TREASURES IN THE DARKNESS

Extending the Early Stage of Lewy Body Dementia, Alzheimer's, and Parkinson's Disease

PAT SNYDER

The information contained in this publication is intended for informational purposes only and should not be construed to be a diagnosis, treatment, regimen, or any other healthcare advice or instruction. The reader should seek his or her own medical or other professional advice, which this publication is not intended to replace or supplement. The author, Pat Snyder, disclaims any responsibility and liability of any kind in connection with the reader's use of the information contained herein. Each reader is advised to make an independent judgment regarding the content and the use of this information.

To Paige
You have been there every day. Your unconditional love
has given us hope and strength.

To John David and Liz
You have given your time, love, and expertise to help
make this book happen.

"And I will give you the treasures of darkness,
and hidden riches of secret places,
that you may know that I, the Lord,
who calls you by your name,
am the God of Israel."
Isaiah 45:3

Contents

Foreword
By Dr. Daniel Kaufer

It is an unexpected privilege and great honor to introduce this book to you. After I had somewhat casually, but earnestly, suggested to Pat Snyder during a routine office visit a while back that she write a book about her experiences as a Lewy Body Dementia caregiver, I had no real expectation of this happening. Yet when the manuscript of this book arrived as an e-mail attachment a few weeks ago, I smiled and said to myself, "Wait a minute, no surprise here. Just another example of Pat Snyder being who she is." Which is to say, a determined, compassionate, insightful, and loving woman who through fate eventually found herself married to a person with Lewy Body Dementia. This book recounts her varied experiences along this journey, offering a vivid portrait of how a person and family grapple with this fairly common, but not widely recognized disorder.

What is Lewy Body Dementia? Lewy Body Dementia is the second most common cause of dementia in adults behind Alzheimer's disease. It is related to Parkinson's disease in that both disorders have microscopic protein deposits (Lewy bodies) in certain areas of the brain. In Parkinson's disease, which was first described almost two hundred years ago as the "shaking palsy," Lewy bodies were thought to only affect parts of the brain that control motor functions, giving rise to motor slowing, stiffness, and a resting tremor. Remarkably, it has only been in the last few decades that researchers have discovered that Lewy body deposits can affect other parts of the brain as well, giving rise to a wide variety of neurological signs and symptoms. These may include marked fluctuations in attention or arousal level, vivid hallucinations (usually involving seeing children or animals that are not really there or thinking that one's spouse is an imposter), motor slowing and stiffness, and seemingly acting out dreams that may involve thrashing about, combativeness, and possible injury to a bed partner. The latter sign, called REM sleep behavior disorder, may appear years or even decades before cognitive and motor signs appear.

Although Lewy Body Dementia was first defined in 1996 (then referred to as "dementia with Lewy bodies"), 40 percent or more of individuals with Parkinson's disease will eventually develop dementia and other features of Lewy Body Dementia. Although individuals with either initial cognitive difficulties (dementia with Lewy bodies) or initial motor dysfunction with subsequently developing dementia (Parkinson's disease dementia) start out differently, eventually the two disorders become virtually indistinguishable clinically and pathologically. The term "Lewy Body Dementia" includes both types of clinical presentations and has important shared treatment implications. In general, individuals with Lewy Body Dementia are exquisitely sensitive to certain types of medications, particularly those that block the brain chemical acetylcholine. Diphenhydramine (Benadryl) is widely used as an over-the-counter sleep aid or cold/allergy remedy and is very strongly anticholinergic, which can provoke confusion and hallucinations. By contrast, medications that are commonly used to treat cognitive symptoms in Alzheimer's disease, such as rivastigmine (Exelon), galantamine (Razadyne), or donepezil (Aricept) may also be useful in treating Lewy Body

Dementia. Neuroleptic or "typical" antipsychotic agents used to treat agitated or psychotic behaviors in schizophrenia (e.g., haloperidol) are sometimes used to treat similar symptoms in Alzheimer's disease, where evidence suggests they may slightly increase the risk of stroke or death. This is also true in Lewy Body Dementia, but additional caution is needed due to the risk of provoking a "neuroleptic sensitivity" reaction, which entails marked alterations in cognitive and motor functioning that often requires hospitalization. At present, it is generally believed that quetiapine (Seroquel) is the safest medication to use in treating marked agitated or psychotic behavior in Lewy Body Dementia patients. Other "atypical" antipsychotic agents such as risperidone (Risperdal) or olanzapine (Zyprexa) are more likely to provoke a sensitivity reaction than quetiapine, but are generally less risky than haloperidol. More research is needed to identify safe and better therapies.

As so poignantly illustrated in this book, greater knowledge and understanding of a complex medical disorder can make it more manageable in myriad ways. First, "knowing the enemy" can offer a sense of control that may otherwise be elusive. The Lewy Body Dementia Association (LBDA—Web site lbda. org) is the primary advocacy group for Lewy Body Dementias and offers a wide range of educational and support services for affected individuals and families, as well as physicians and other health care providers. A caregiver survey conducted on the LBDA Web site involving over nine hundred respondents reported that on average, over three physicians were consulted for a diagnostic evaluation before a diagnosis of Lewy Body Dementia was made. Almost 25 percent of individuals that were eventually diagnosed with Lewy Body Dementia were initially diagnosed as having a mental disorder. Greater education and public awareness will help affected individuals and their families get more prompt diagnosis and treatment. In the fall of 2011, Lewy Body Dementia became accepted into the Social Security Administration's Compassionate Allowance program with the help of vigorous lobbying efforts by LBDA. This determination will streamline the process of obtaining disability benefits for individuals with Lewy Body Dementia.

While scientific research pushes the boundaries of diagnostic testing and therapeutic treatments for Lewy Body Dementia forward, approximately 1.3 million individuals and their families are currently dealing with various stages of Lewy Body Dementia. Many of these individuals have yet to be and may never be diagnosed. While it is important for primary care physicians to be able to recognize the cardinal features of Lewy Body Dementia and understand basic principles of treatment, these disorders can be challenging to manage even by experienced specialists. The multiple array of symptoms and signs, and their evolution over time leads to a great deal of variability from individual case to case. Some patients with Lewy Body Dementia may respond quite dramatically to available treatments, whereas others may respond only modestly, if at all. Overall, it has been my experience that most cases of "dramatic improvement" have involved removing one or more medications that were causing or exacerbating prominent clinical symptoms. These are the cases that absolutely should not be missed. This underscores the importance of obtaining a comprehensive diagnostic evaluation by a knowledgeable medical professional and following up at regular intervals. Of course, even the most experienced doctors make mistakes and, in some cases, never know because the patient doesn't return to see them. We can only hope to minimize the number of errors we make and learn from them.

As illustrated in this book, probably the single most important factor that colors the experience of being a *person* affected by

Lewy Body Dementia, or being a loved one caring for a person with Lewy Body Dementia, is attitude. A positive, supportive, and optimistic attitude is the most potent weapon we currently have against degenerative brain disorders such as Lewy Body Dementia to fuel hope and motivate participation in research.

Daniel Kaufer, MD

Division Chief, Cognitive Neurology & Memory Disorders
Director, UNC Memory Disorders Program
Associate Professor, Neurology
Director, Carolina Alzheimer's Network

Foreword
By Dr. Terry Ledford

It seems that every stage of life is accompanied by a dream. Children dream of the perceived independence of adolescence. Teenagers dream of the "real" independence of adulthood. When we find that perfect partner, we dream of the perfect marriage. We dream of having children, and then the future experiences and relationships with those children. In middle age, we dream of travel, taking well-earned time off, growing older gracefully and in good health. We all make plans. We all create dreams.

Unfortunately, dreams are sometimes interrupted. The diagnosis of a catastrophic illness such as Lewy Body Dementia can shatter such dreams in one deafening sentence, even when it is spoken in compassionate tones. The patient and the family go through shock, numbness, confusion, anger, depression, and grief. The blow can send one reeling, and regaining one's footing can take time.

To say that one experiences blessings in an illness sounds strange. To imagine that a person, a marriage, or a family can grow in the midst of a catastrophe seems unthinkable, yet it often occurs. Like gold brought to the surface by an earthquake, blessings can be revealed by the worst of events. I have seen this happen as I have accompanied John and Pat on this journey. I have seen them grow in understanding. I have seen them more fully realize and communicate the deep love they had always felt for each other. As they encountered each challenge, I saw them work more as a team. I saw them experience blessings.

I have had the honor of being John and Pat's counselor as they confronted Lewy Body Dementia and the adjustments required by that disease. I truly do feel honored to have been allowed to share this intense and personal time in their lives.

In the pages that follow, Pat Snyder has shared, with a tenacious honesty, the heart of a caregiver. She has revealed the struggles of a family attempting to understand and cope with catastrophic illness. Out of their experiences with the medical system, she offers wise advice concerning the need to become one's own healthcare advocate. She has also shared the growth and blessings revealed, as she and John have walked through this path life has given them.

Each journey will be different, but I believe that the reader will find much to relate to in this brave couple's story. I believe this book will provide a sense of shared experience for many. It is always comforting to know that one is not alone.

Dr. Terry Ledford
Psychologist
President, Woodridge Psychological Associates

Introduction

This is a book for early stage Lewy Body Dementia caregivers. Lewy Body Dementia (LBD) includes elements of both Alzheimer's and Parkinson's diseases, so it may be helpful for the caregivers of those patients as well.

In this book, I address ways to adjust and cope with the diagnosis while your loved one is still in the early stage of the disease. I share things I did well and things I handled poorly. When my husband, John, was diagnosed with LBD in 2007, my quest was to find anything and everything that would prolong this stage of the disease to enrich life as long as possible. Like Alzheimer's and Parkinson's, there is no cure for this progressive disease (but always hope for a cure). Prolonging your current stage is your best and only option. As my husband's neurologist says, our primary goal is to "preserve personhood."

I have written this book because my husband's neurologist, Dr. Daniel Kaufer, told me that I was doing the things that had made a difference in extending stage one LBD for John. He told me I needed to share what I was doing with others because it might help them. I am not a medical expert—just a caregiver who wants to do all I can to make a difference. My advice should not be taken as any form of medical expertise. It is simply what has worked for us and may not work for others.

If you are reading this, it is likely that your family has been hit with the devastating diagnosis of an incurable, progressive disease. You are probably still reeling from that. I understand. I have been there.

My first word of comfort to you is that you will not stay in this emotional place forever. You will get through this. It may take time, but you will adjust and get a grip on life as it now must be.

If the disease is still in the early stage, there are things you can do for your loved one and for yourself that will make a difference in the quality of your lives every day. You may actually find something good in the midst of all this. I know that sounds crazy right now, but it is possible. What you decide to do and how you choose to react can have an impact on the reality that you now face.

LBD is different for each patient and family, and that is one of the reasons it is so hard to diagnose and deal with. But there are some common characteristics of the cognitive, emotional, psychological, and physical symptoms that the caregiver can address to help alleviate the impact of this disease, especially in the early stage.

By extending the early stage of LBD as long as possible, you gain good times with each other. You give the researchers more time to find what could be a turning point solution for some of the symptoms or even a reversal of the disease. So much progress has been made in research and treatment in recent years for both Alzheimer's and Parkinson's diseases. The good news for LBD patients is that many of those medicines are more effective for the treatment of LBD symptoms. Most importantly, the personhood of your loved one can be preserved and even enhanced in the early stage by some choices you can control.

This book tells our story and shares those tips that helped us in practical ways to not just cope, but even to grow as human beings and as a family on this journey that none of us wanted to take.

TREASURES IN THE DARKNESS

1
Diagnosis Doomsday
June 8, 2007

"**M**om, Dad has Lewy Body Disease," Paige said. My daughter was on the phone with me. I was at home, sick in bed, unable to make the appointment with the neurologist at a prestigious research hospital. He was supposed to give my husband and me some answers or some direction about what had been going on in his body for such a long time.

Over a year of intensive searching for answers to what was happening to John had led to more questions with more potential solutions. But new problems kept creeping up, or old ones reappearing, after trying multiple medicines and techniques. Over time, we had seen ten different doctors, who were frustrating to deal with because they were too busy to really listen; they could see only part of the problem; they just did not know what to do; or they tried hard to help, but were stumped.

John's medical file at home had grown to over two inches thick, and his symptoms fit all manner of possible diagnoses. When I had asked John's primary care doctor if John should retire, she had said, "No, Pat, this could turn on a dime."

"What in the world is Lewy Body Disease?" I said, unknowingly resting on my last piece of solid emotional ground for many months to come.

"I have a lot of information they gave me to share with you, Mom. But the bottom line is that it acts like a combination of Alzheimer's and Parkinson's."

"What? A combination of Alzheimer's and Parkinson's? How can there be such a monster out there?" My voice was soft, but my heart felt like it had stopped. The world froze.

ଊଠଷ

Paige and John had left the hospital complex feeling hopeless. Paige tried to get her dad to stay with her until she could contact me, but all he wanted to do was to get home.

"He wants to get home to you as fast as he can, Mom. I could not stop him. He was weaving all over the road at one point."

It felt like a quiet horror edged with denial and doubt that this could really be happening.

"What did the doctor say? Aren't there any medicines that can help him? Wasn't anything prescribed?" I said.

Paige continued, "I have notes and a lot of details to share with you. They recommend a Mediterranean diet and exercise. They urged us to go ahead and plan for you two to move into an assisted living center setting, one of those communities that has levels of care, to try to cushion the financial impact. It is important that he not get sick because he will get worse."

"Now? Your dad doesn't seem to be in need of that kind of thing yet. Wasn't there anything else they could do to help?" I said.

"Well, the doctor said it was wise to plan ahead and the nurse clearly recommended it again after he left, saying that this was often financially devastating to a family. She said it was what she would do," said Paige.

"Good grief! How in the world can you have both Alzheimer's and Parkinson's? Surely there is some treatment to help the symptoms. Is there any follow up?"

"They said Dad was to come back in six months and have an appointment with the nurse practitioner. She has all kinds of helpful information about support groups and kinds of community help that I need to give you. There are some papers here."

I was confused. "When is he going to see the doctor again?"

"I don't know. They just said to come back and see the nurse practitioner in six months."

"What was this doctor like? Was he sure about the diagnosis?" By this time in my journey into the land of US medicine, I was skeptical about Doctor Number Eleven.

"He was immaculately dressed, very neat, very intelligent, cool, and professional looking. You could tell he was taking in every detail by the way his eyes scanned Dad's body and movements. He was clearly thinking and evaluating the whole time he was in the exam room. He was watching every move and analyzing everything, like when you are buying a new car. He was very interested in the bear Dad thought he saw behind the house. He said it was a hallucination. The nurse said that he was correct in his diagnoses about 97 percent of the time and that we had come to the right place.

"He was obviously very bright, Mom. Do you want me to call John David? (her brother)"

"Yes. I have to process all this. How can there be such a monster out there?"

As Paige and John left the clinic, the tone was doomsday. Paige later said it felt like, "This is going downhill fast, and Dad's days are numbered." John later said he just felt totally without hope.

2
Hunt for an Answer before Doomsday

L et me take you back through what had happened leading up to this doomsday diagnosis.

For more than two decades, John had sleep apnea, and then he developed REM sleep disorder. That went on for about fifteen years, gradually getting worse over time.

Sometime in 2000, I started to notice slight changes in John. There was nothing specific that I can recall except that his eye color actually changed from blue to gray. He did not seem to have the energy he needed. He had gone to one of those health screening events that pass through our community every now and then. There appeared to be a blockage in his carotid artery, and something seemed to be in his neck that was suspicious.

Upon further checking with his primary care doctor and follow-up tests, the artery blockage seemed to be about normal for his age, but the growth was not. He had a fast-growing tumor on his thyroid gland. The surgeon noted that John seemed "flat in affect" when we visited his office for a consultation about possible surgery.

I was adamant that any growth needed to be removed immediately. The thought of anything suspicious growing inside

John was shocking and scary to me. The surgeon told us that it might be treatable with medicines, but John agreed to the surgery, probably because of my strong reaction and fears.

When John came out of surgery in the spring of 2001, his first words to me were, "This was a big mistake."

Based on what I have learned from other caregivers since then, his words might have been prophetic. For some sufferers of LBD, the trigger event seems to be a surgery.

After the thyroid was removed, John had to begin thyroid hormone replacement therapy. Strangely, though, the surgeon did not recommend that he see an endocrinologist. John's internist at the time prescribed the hormones. John never fully came back to his presurgical "normal" in my opinion. We were always trying to tweak his hormonal levels to get his energy level restored. His voice volume was low after surgery and never came back, but his eye color did.

In spite of all this, we were able to enjoy the active, normal routines of our work lives. I was teaching, and John was running a successful law practice after retiring from the district attorney's office. We took wonderful vacations to Europe each year.

While in Italy in July 2002, John asked me if I would like to come and work as his office manager and paralegal at the law office. I was a little nervous about it, but also thrilled about getting to have the same schedule and working together. Since I had always had an interest in law and had been accepted to UNC Law School just after college graduation, the thought of being in the midst of his world for a season became more and more appealing.

We had a discussion of how we would run the office if I were there and how we would approach it. We decided on a low-key style of moving gradually toward retirement and reducing the types of cases he would take bit by bit. I promised to control his schedule to allow for more vacation time as we eased toward retirement.

When we returned from Italy, the details fell into place. Looking back, it was a blessing that I went to work in John's office when I did. For years afterward, life consisted of full and happy days. We shared our work and took great vacations. Both children got married six months apart, and our first grandson, Michael, was born in 2005. All through this, we had to keep tweaking the thyroid hormone replacement to keep John at his best. Hints of something that was not quite right nagged us.

After a while, John's caseload began to demand more support staff than I could provide by myself. We added another paralegal to his law office to make sure he had what he needed and was prepared for cases. John began to lean more and more on that support over time.

By mid-August 2006, we had moved to a new primary care physician who was a great listener. Doctor Lori Dickson was the fourth doctor to see John since 2000. She began attacking John's various symptoms as they became obvious. She agreed with the family's conclusion that John might have some level of depression. He was withdrawn at family gatherings. Since he also had peripheral neuropathy (nerve damage that causes numbness and pain in hands or feet) in his feet, she prescribed Cymbalta because it would address both the neuropathy and the depression. She also gave him testosterone hormone replacement when blood tests showed that to be low. John's symptoms improved. He had more energy and was more engaged across the board.

In mid-September 2006, John was at the courthouse when he felt some chest pain. I insisted that he go to the hospital. He was admitted for an overnight stay and had some erratic blood pressure readings while there. The hospitalist, who was doctor number five since 2000, prescribed a blood pressure medication, but found no signs of heart problems. After that, John went through a period in which his blood pressure fluctuated significantly. It took six months of adjusting blood pressure medications before it settled to acceptable and consistent levels.

During this period each issue was being addressed separately while I and his doctor tried to put it all together. With multiple medical conditions that included his thyroid, depression, peripheral neuropathy, asthma, sleep disorders, and blood pressure, this puzzle was getting complicated. Medicines were being added and tweaked, and John would improve and then have bad days.

In spite of all this, John was still enjoying his law practice. When I asked his primary care doctor if John should retire, she said, "No, Pat, this could turn on a dime."

I was researching almost every day online, hunting for answers and trying to get at the cause of each symptom as it arose and fluctuated in and out of our lives. John seemed to appreciate my research but did not participate in it. There was a gradual and frustrating decline in John's ability to initiate activity at work or at home, to process information, to write neatly, to focus his attention. But it fluctuated. At times he was sharp as a tack and on point. Out of nowhere, he would drop into a "bad day" or a bad afternoon.

Late in 2006, we made two traumatic visits to the ER for constipation. Those were two very rough days. John had a long-term lack of thirst awareness. He would even seem to be proud of going long stretches of time without water. After the ER visits, John drank at least six to eight glasses of water every day. Even then, though, I was reminding him to do it. The increased water consumption seemed to address the constipation issue.

In November 2006, on one of his bad days, he had a minor traffic accident pulling out of a parking space and almost hit my car at the same time. I had to back up fast to avoid being hit by him. His doctor ordered a CAT scan that day, which showed only a small spot on one of his endocrine glands that seemed unimportant. Otherwise, his brain looked healthy.

We requested a referral to an endocrinologist to pursue thyroid issues, low testosterone levels, and that small spot. In December 2006, there were two visits with the endocrinologist, who was doctor number six. A test revealed that John's pituitary gland was not functioning.

On Christmas Eve 2006, two days before his second visit with the endocrinologist, John and I were at Paige's house. John came downstairs profoundly confused. He could not fix his own cup of coffee and had stiff, awkward body movements. His brain was obviously not working right for some reason. We were frightened. After eating, he became euphoric and went into a silly state that lasted for hours. I called the endocrinologist, and he recommended that John see a psychiatrist and ordered an MRI. A few hours later, John was back to normal, so we all assumed that he had mixed up his medicines when he took them before coming downstairs.

On the trip home from the research triangle area on December 28, I had a revelation during our discussion over lunch. John did something as we talked that rang a bell for me as a former educator. As we sat at lunch, I recognized that he had just behaved like students I had taught who had attention deficit disorder. At home, we listened to tapes that described classic symptoms and experiences of those with ADD. John related to these and shared memories of issues he had dealt with as a young student.

In January 2007, I witnessed John being confused in the courtroom. A young attorney came over to assist us, and I was able to take some simple actions to get John refocused. It turned out well, but I was shaken by what I saw. The dilemma about when to close the law office was intensifying as I saw for myself how this could play out in the courtroom.

We loved our work and had clients who needed the extra attention our staff provided. Knowing when to stop practicing was getting easier to see, in spite of what John's doctor had said. There were beginning to be too many symptoms.

Six days later we were at home, and John thought he saw a bear in the woods behind our house. It turned out to be a tree stump and did look like a bear, but he called the police before telling me. I looked out the window and saw two policemen walking in our backyard with John. When he came back inside the house and told me what he had done, I fell onto the bed crying, "What have you done? You work with these people!" After a while, we talked and decided that John needed a month's medical leave to search intensively for answers to what was happening to him.

January 2007 was a busy month. John's blood pressure continued to fluctuate wildly. He had begun taking a statin, which a seventh doctor prescribed when Dr. Dickson was unavailable for a period of time. We discontinued the statin in June upon discovering it could conflict with his thyroid hormone replacement. This is another example of how a doctor can step into the picture, look at one or two symptoms, and cause more problems or confuse the issue for a patient.

Later in January, John had an MRI, which showed no issues in the brain. He visited a psychiatrist twice, who ordered blood tests and gave a possible diagnosis of neurovascular problems with complications of hypertension. This eighth physician recommended John see a neurologist with likelihood of an MRA test, which provides pictures of blood vessels that may reveal reduced blood flow. The psychiatrist also diagnosed John as having ADD, but said John could not receive treatment for it until vascular issues were ruled out.

So we saw a ninth doctor, a local neurologist, who suspected the endocrine system was the culprit. She agreed with me that dopamine might be involved in a number of John's symptoms. In order to rule out vascular causes, she ordered a sonogram of the carotid arteries and MRA of the neck and head.

In February 2007, John had the tests ordered by the neurologist, revisited the endocrinologist for test interpretation, discovered that his testosterone replacement hormone needed to be doubled, still had fluctuating blood pressure, and began treatment for ADD with Concerta. He felt more focused and alert after this.

In March, John returned to work with a reduced workload. We adjusted his work calendar according to his symptoms, changing appointments and court days as needed. His blood pressure was still all over the map. The trajectory was not positive in terms of his alertness and ability to focus, and the symptoms kept rearing their ugly heads over and over again.

On April 2, 2007, we made the decision to retire and close the office after an out of town judge spoke to our resident Superior Court judge about concerns he had after watching John in court. It was getting harder and harder to schedule around his bad days and give John the support he needed to represent clients well in court. We felt the medical solution was just around the corner, and our doctor agreed with us, but the battle had become too much.

Since we planned to eventually move closer to our children, we thought it might be wise to find a doctor in the research triangle area of North Carolina. The area is rich with medical resources. Paige helped us locate an internist with a good reputation, and we saw him in May. As doctor number ten, he referred us to Doctor Number Eleven, who diagnosed John in early June 2007 as having LBD.

The problem with LBD, as I have come to understand it, is that it presents an array of symptoms that can vary hugely between different patients. Then, on top of that, the cognitive abilities like attention, alertness, or confusion fluctuate, so that some symptoms come and go for short or long periods of time. It also mimics, in part, several other diseases or conditions. Plus, LBD does not happen in a vacuum. Other medical conditions can occur with symptom overlap. Medications can have side effects or conflict with other medicines, causing confusion of symptoms. It was maddening getting our diagnosis.

On the diagnosis journey, we saw twelve doctors: three primary care physicians, two internists, one endocrinologist, one psychiatrist, one surgeon, one hospitalist, and three neurologists. There were several ER doctors as well.

3
After Diagnosis—
Research LBD

I cannot remember exactly what happened when John reached home after his LBD diagnosis with Doctor Number Eleven. Maybe it was too emotional, and I have blocked it out. I know that we held each other and cried and talked about how bowled over we were by it. I remember feeling a dazed, numb shock and being driven to find out more. I tend to be a delayed reactor and a problem solver by nature. When I am presented with a bad event, I start thinking about how I can fix it, how I can get control of it somehow, but this time the problem was overpowering.

John had already given notice of his retirement from his law practice to all who needed to know in April, two months before this doctor appointment. Before the LBD diagnosis, I had a lot of work as his office manager to finish closing his office. Now I had another mission.

Every day and night I was on the computer looking for more information about LBD and for a good neurologist who might give us a second opinion about his diagnosis and possible treatments.

I was also looking for a house near our children. Both of them live in the same area of North Carolina, about three to four hours away from us, near excellent hospitals and specialists. Doctor Number Eleven had made us all feel like we needed to move, and the sooner the better.

4
Find a House, Find a House, Find a House

With an eye toward retirement, starting around 2005, I had started a leisurely review of homes that John and I might like if we moved to the Research Triangle area of North Carolina to be near our children and future grandchildren. It was fun and stimulating to dream about starting a new life in a place where we had both gone to college and graduate school, where we had met and fallen in love.

Our daughter, Paige, and her husband, Dave, announced in early 2005 that our first grandbaby was on the way and due around Thanksgiving. Paige and I talked about how great it would be if John and I could retire to the Triangle area. We could enjoy more grandbaby time and give her some free time by babysitting, so she could work on the administrative side of their basketball scouting service. We were both excited about that.

On October 3, 2005, Paige had an emergency C-section to deliver our first grandson, Michael, eight weeks early. She developed postpartum depression, and I ended up staying in Wake Forest with her family for five weeks to help as she recovered and Michael started life as a preemie. During that time, it made sense that Paige could benefit from having John and me close by to give her support as a new mom while her husband, Dave, who is a basketball scout, traveled many days each month.

By June 2007, when Dr. Number Eleven gave the diagnosis of LBD and the dire prediction of our need for extra support, my fears kicked in big time. House hunting for a place closer to our family moved from a pleasant option to an obsession.

I remember spending all my evening hours at the computer looking at real estate in the triangle area and searching for what we needed at an affordable price. I was convinced that if I worked hard enough, I could solve this problem and come up with a solution that would help us all. Friends have told me that they were worried about me because I became so intense about it.

We were almost four hours away from our kids by car, over two hundred miles. It was five hours from my mother and other family in eastern North Carolina. We had no relatives in Rutherford County, where we lived. Our house was wonderful, our yard was lovely and peaceful, but I felt stranded away from family. John was happy where we were but open to moving.

All I could think about was finding a way that we could affordably move into a much higher priced real estate market and live close to my children. I was running on fear and adrenaline. I knew that LBD patients needed familiarity, that moving could exacerbate John's symptoms, but fear of being alone weighed more heavily on my mind. My friends and family tried to get me to take it easy and go more slowly, but I was on a mission and would not be deterred.

My good friend of many years, Beth, was trying her hand at real estate in the Triangle area at the time. I enlisted her help in trying to find the right house that would meet John's future needs and be close to the kids. On more than one occasion, I was ready to make an offer when the house would sell right out from under my nose. I now see that as God's protection, but at the time it was frustrating.

Finally, right around the time of John's diagnosis, I found it. It was pretty, in a great neighborhood with convenient shopping nearby, and the price was fabulous because it was on the verge of foreclosure. I had done my homework and knew that similar houses on that block had sold for tens of thousands of dollars more than the asking price.

When I stepped in the door, I knew immediately that this was the house. My arms tingled and were covered with chill bumps as I walked inside. The plan was open and flowing with lots of space for all our stuff. It was a two story, but with the low price and lots of extra space, we could afford to have a small elevator installed and make modifications to allow John to easily navigate inside and out. John liked it, too.

Another plus in my mind was that it was located five doors down from Paige's house. Our mutual support of each other would be so simplified. Paige had told me earlier that Dave had said, "Do whatever it takes," when I had asked about moving, so I assumed everyone was on board.

I knew someone was about to make an offer on the house, so I told Beth to draw up our offer. Little did I know at that time that a meltdown was just around the corner for me, John, and the whole family.

5
Meltdown

It was Father's Day weekend a couple of weeks after the diagnosis, and John and I were staying in Wake Forest with our daughter and son-in-law. Paige was to fly to England the following Tuesday for a week's visit with a friend. John and I had agreed to keep our grandson, Michael, for her and Dave while she was gone.

I was so excited about making the offer on the house and wanted to tell everybody at the same time. John, Paige, Dave, John David, and his wife, Liz, were all in Paige and Dave's family room when I told them how excited I was about the house down the street.

Dave's reaction was not what I expected. He was not in favor of us moving down the street. I was stunned. My impression was that they had supported us in a move nearby, but Dave's anger conveyed another story.

To be fair, the offer on the house happened quickly due to foreclosure pressures and another offer being made at the same time. Dave had been out of town as this all came together and pretty much came home from the road to a life-changing curve ball. And Paige was trying to meet everyone's needs while reeling from her dad's diagnosis.

Dave and I loudly exchanged some words I cannot remember. Paige tried to get him to sit down. John David said something to the effect that Dave and I were talking past each other, and neither of us was listening to the emotional needs the other was expressing. John said something like this now looked like a bad idea.

I was expecting harmonious family unity in these moments, and what I was getting was the opposite. It felt like they were not agreeing with me. My little vision of everyone being happy about such a good real estate find that would get us established close by did not match up with reality at all.

Everyone got up to go eat dinner in the dining room, but I sat alone in the family room in a daze. I could not join them. I felt betrayed by every single one of them. It felt like a black and deep suction downward into myself.

I had to get out of there. I grabbed my car keys and headed toward the door. I saw John David's car was blocking mine, so I went to the dining room and asked him in a dull but firm voice to move his car so I could get out. He tried to comfort me, but I was having none of it. All I wanted was to leave, leave, leave. I remember glancing at his worried face as I pulled out of Paige's driveway.

I pointed the car eastward, heading toward my mother's house. Tears poured down my face, as all my best plans were crashing around me. It felt like all my family had deserted me. I had no more ideas at that point. They had rejected what I thought made perfect sense for everybody.

Now I realize that we were all just raw.

As I tore down the narrow country road toward my mother's house, an hour away in Rocky Mount, I screamed over and over as loud as I could, "I want my mama!" I beat on the steering wheel, screamed, and cried. It was primal. The last straw of over a year's worth of straws had landed on me, and I broke.

By the time I reached Mama's house, I felt washed out, empty, and exhausted. All I could do was sit on the edge of her couch in her family room and stare at the floor. I asked her to call Robin, my sister, and told them both what had happened. They were totally and gently supportive, which made a huge difference.

Later in the evening, John David called, probably checking to see if I had gone to Mama's house. Both Mama and Robin talked to him and explained my distress. They defended me strongly and told John David he was going to have to step up and be the "man of the family," that I really needed him now. Based on what I had told them, they assumed I had been deeply wronged and let down. Their defense of me felt good, and it gave me strength when I needed it. I told them to tell him that I was "done," not clarifying what that meant. I ended up staying there for a couple of days.

Paige called on Sunday and asked if I was still going to keep Michael and to say they had arranged for Dave's parents to keep him if I could not. She desperately needed to get away herself to get a break from all the drama our family had been through in the past couple of years and especially in the past two weeks. She was carrying a heavy emotional load.

I was in no shape to keep a nineteen-month-old, so they decided to take Michael to Dave's parents while Paige was in England.

I went back to Paige's to get John, and we both went back to Mama's to spend the night before heading home. I did not look anyone in the eyes at that time and, frankly, did not want to see them at all.

But John was another story. That was when I realized the trauma my meltdown and quick departure had caused him. He looked dazed and worried. Later that night, he told me he thought I was leaving him. I reassured him that I was not leaving, just deeply hurt and reeling from all my plans being rejected so abruptly and unexpectedly on the heels of hearing the diagnosis we had heard a few days earlier. I told him that I wanted to take a week or two away, which I did a couple of weeks later, just to recharge from everything—visiting friends and family for some down time.

I said, "Don't worry. I am sticking this out with you. I just need a break for a little while to get my energy back. I am not going anywhere."

6
A Second Opinion Needed

After the initial diagnosis of LBD, my memory of what came next is not clear. I suppose the shock of it all has blurred what happened and what I was feeling at the time. I remember John saying that Doctor Number Eleven looked him in the eye and said, "You need to retire now."

Even though we had already made that decision, it was the first time any medical professional had told either of us to do that. The closing date already established was June 30, and we already had most of the work done to bring it to closure on the Superior Court date at the end of June. The doctor's words simply solidified that commitment.

I also remember searching the Internet for hours every day and night, seeking information about LBD and possible treatments as well as current research on Alzheimer's and Parkinson's medicines. I needed background information for greater understanding of what we were dealing with and what may be coming at us. We had no medical advocate to turn to. There was also a question of whether the diagnosis was correct because of so much conflicting and confusing information and possible causes for the long list of symptoms. We could never know for sure how capable each doctor was or whether he or she was an effective listener in such a complex situation. LBD is a bear to diagnose.

In late June 2007, I was looking on the Lewy Body Dementia Association Web site, lbda.org, for any helpful information. I ran across the name of Dr. Daniel Kaufer, who was listed as a member of the Scientific Advisory Council. As I read brief biographical information about him, I was surprised to see that he was practicing at UNC Memorial Hospital in Chapel Hill, our alma mater. I went to the UNC Web site where I found confirmation that LBD was a primary area of interest to him. His picture also reminded me of my daddy, which I took to be a "Go-for-it!" sign.

I was on the phone to his office as soon as I could get to it. Karen, his assistant, was warm and helpful. When I told her the purpose of my call and gave her a brief history of our situation, she said, "You have come to the right place. This is exactly what Dr. Kaufer does. He will be able to help you see if you have the right diagnosis." But she told me there was a likely waiting time of about six months to see the doctor.

I asked Karen if we could be put on a waiting list. I told her we would drop everything and could be there within three to four hours if anyone cancelled and would happily do so to be able to see Dr. Kaufer as soon as possible. She assured me that we would be called if anyone cancelled, and a few days later Karen called with a July 17 appointment for John.

This time, I wanted all the family in place to see and hear everything that happened during the visit with Dr. Kaufer. I did not want to miss or forget anything that might be helpful. So our daughter, Paige, and our son, John David, came along with John and me on that first visit.

To prepare for it, I consolidated all the history beginning with the exam that identified the thyroid tumor in 2000 down to the initial diagnosis by Doctor Number Eleven. It was three pages long. I had a summary sheet of all John's medicines with a symbol system identifying impacts each one had made on his symptoms. There were also test results and the film and CDs from the CAT scan, MRI, carotid artery sonogram, and MRA tests. I spent hours gathering and consolidating all this information for Dr. Kaufer, who was doctor number twelve in our journey.

Just before John's appointment, I was nervous but hopeful that we might find out that John's diagnosis was wrong. It felt good to know I was walking in with our children, who would be able to give us support and also answer questions if needed. It also felt good that I had done my own homework in preparing so much information for Dr. Kaufer. That gave me confidence that he would be able to see all the details to solve this long, complicated mystery. I do not remember any conversations with John the night before the appointment. There was an undercurrent of pins and needles among us.

7
First Visit with Dr. Kaufer

On July 17, 2007, all four Snyders entered the UNC neurology department with varying degrees of nervousness and anticipation of a new point of view about what was happening to John.

I was armed with my three page presentation for Dr. Kaufer, who was the twelfth doctor (excluding ER visits) to see John, confident that I had the bases covered in terms of the history of our journey. I was sure Dr. Kaufer would be impressed and appreciative as other doctors had been for my diligence and attention to detail.

John David had his laptop ready to go. I had asked him to help me remember what was said and done during our appointment, but was surprised when he showed up with his computer, which he opened upon getting settled into the exam room.

Dr. Kaufer stuck his head in the door first, smiled, and entered with an assistant. He was dressed neatly and had a brisk, confident air about him. He asked in a firm and inquisitive tone, "John, why are you here?" I do not remember John's answer.

I handed him the stack of papers I had prepared and said something to the effect that we had been on a long journey and hoped this would help him to see what we were really dealing with. Dr. Kaufer glanced at the top page and then tossed them all to the table at his side and said, "So it's complicated."

My jaw dropped. My mind went blank.

He continued in conversation with John that was a blur to me as I struggled to focus and think clearly. I did not want to miss an opportunity to give information that would help with a correct diagnosis. But I was stunned and beginning to feel angry with this guy.

I thought, "The nerve of him to dismiss all my work just like that! How dare he do that! He is going to miss something really important that he needs to know for a correct diagnosis."

I answered a number of his questions, but my mind was in a real muddle at that point. When he finally asked me what the three biggest changes had been in John in the last five years, my mind pulled a blank. My answers were not really on point, I think, because I could not make myself concentrate. The pressure of this long medical journey came crashing down on me full force in this exam room when I most needed to think clearly.

About five minutes into the appointment, Dr. Kaufer said that he can usually figure out what is going on, but he was having trouble figuring that out with John. I am not sure if my loss of clarity added to that.

Thirty minutes in, he still was piecing the details together as I was beginning to think more clearly, give more information, and answer questions more to my own satisfaction.

We ended up spending more than two hours with Dr. Kaufer and his assistant. Dr. Kaufer was focused on John, getting him to answer questions and perform motor actions. He read test results, looked at films, probed us with questions, and had his assistant test John. John David was taking notes all the time, and John, Paige, and John David were all adding their insights as needed, especially when they saw me struggling to share all that had happened. I was so glad that they were with us. It was the first time all of us had been in the room with John and a doctor, and I now realize how important that was for many reasons. They could fill in obvious gaps of information that John and I missed. They could remember and even record what was being said for future reference. They could give the eye contact across the room that made being there bearable.

Dr. Kaufer tried more than once to joke with me about my need to get things down on paper and had me fill out information sheets about caregiving that gave him data he needed to help in his diagnosis. His light joking only increased my irritation at that point. I felt dismissed, demeaned, and discarded. I was not a Kaufer fan.

Paige said I looked like a mouse trapped in a corner. I was used to being the bearer of vital and detailed information, and this doctor had taken over with a different approach. As the twelfth physician to evaluate John marched on in his procedures, I sat there feeling insulted, rejected, dazed, and angry. But mostly, I was scared to death that our best chance to get to the bottom of John's problem was lying on a side table in written form, and this doctor would not even look at it. There was so much that had happened to John that I wanted him to see. What if he missed a key detail that would unravel the mystery?

This doctor wanted to ask his own questions and avoid the clutter of too much information, but I could not see that at the time. He was also trying to jar me out of my rut and get me to listen to him. His intention was good, but I interpreted his brusque style as lacking in understanding or compassion. He seemed to be a selective listener when I would point to the pages I brought and say, "It is all right there." After I repeated that to him, Dr. Kaufer finally picked up my report and keyed in on the list of symptoms. That helped me to relax somewhat.

After persistently digging for facts, Dr. Kaufer did confirm the LBD diagnosis, but said John had a "very mild case." Technically John did not meet the full criteria and would be classified with a mild cognitive impairment.

He told John that he was too healthy to qualify for any studies. After looking at the films, he told John, "You have a beautiful brain." It was a wonderful shock to hear some good news. The feeling was somewhat like a roller coaster ride with bad news of the LBD diagnosis, but good news of his current status.

He also told us that what John had was very treatable. He said it was progressive, but the symptoms, just like with diabetes, were treatable.

Dr. Kaufer laid out a game plan for treatment that began with addressing John's quality of sleep issues. Memory and motor issues were not a major problem right now, and his current medicines were already addressing mood and other issues.

At this point, I agreed and connected with Dr. Kaufer's logic. He was going to the source, the beginning point of the problem, by helping John's brain get enough quality sleep so that it could restore and heal itself for the demands of the next day. I started to like what he had to say more. He was making good sense.

He also kept emphasizing that we do only one thing at a time. He insisted on a small change with time for it to have an impact and then a reassessment of John's needs. Our pattern had been too many changes too fast, and he was trying to break this pattern because it added to the confusion instead of leading to solutions. It would also mean that I could slow down in my frantic search for answers. But I did not understand this until later. All I could feel right then was anger with a tinge of hope.

What I did not realize, until the four of us were walking out of the hospital, was that something important had happened at that appointment.

I was walking behind John, Paige, and John David, having a fine little pity party about my papers being tossed to one side. I was seething about what a jerk Dr. Kaufer was for dismissing my work and arrogantly tossing it on that table. I decided I did not like him at all. I could feel my face burning with humiliation and indignation.

Then I started hearing what the other three Snyders were saying to each other. I looked at their body language, especially at how John was walking with a much more confident stride than he had used when we entered the building. They were all so happy! They were laughing and enjoying the moment together while they made comments of relief and approval about the appointment.

I could see that they were in one place emotionally while I was in another. I decided to be quiet. Maybe they were more in touch with something good that I had just missed.

Then John said it. "I have hope."

The kids responded with delighted soft laughter. "Yeah, Dad, so do I. That's good!" said John David. Paige was totally on board with them and responded in kind.

I knew I needed to stay quiet and let them enjoy that moment. I also knew I must be off base and needed to recalibrate my feelings.

8
Adjusting to the Right Doctor

D r. Kaufer's treatment plan of addressing sleep quality first was a bridge for me. It helped me move from skepticism to trust in terms of my caregiver relationship to him as John's neurologist. I was specialist-doctor weary at this point and still wincing from when he tossed aside my papers that included all the background on John's history.

When he said, "Let's work on getting a good night's sleep first," that made sense to me. I wanted to be active in helping to solve that problem because John did not tolerate CPAP therapy at all. Twenty years of poor sleep quality needed addressing in my opinion.

The first symptom of a possible future with LBD might be sleep disorder issues such as REM sleep disorder. Years ago John's feet started to flutter after he drifted off to sleep. At first, I thought it was funny because of the strange and quick movement that appeared out of nowhere.

Over time, movement progressed up his legs and his arms started to jerk some. He would reach out with his hands as if trying to grasp something in thin air, and his face would move to show emotions. He would laugh or talk out loud, obviously involved in conversation with someone in his dream state.

Eventually, he moved to thrashing around, acting out dramatic events of his dreams. Once I told him to wake up when he almost hit me with his arm. I asked him what he was dreaming, and he replied that he was in the middle of a sword fight on a ship. That one was scary and funny at the same time. Another time he thrashed around and fell off the bed, acting out some sort of fight from his dreams. He hit his head on the corner of the nightstand and got a nasty cut and bruise from that adventure.

We joked about how he must be processing all the courtroom battles symbolically in his dreams. But eventually we had to start sleeping in separate places just so I could get a good night's sleep and not get hit by mistake.

When Dr. Kaufer targeted John's sleep issues as his first line of attack, I was happy. I knew that the brain needs to have deep restorative sleep to clean itself out, refresh itself, and process events and emotions from the day. The neurologist's method made a lot of sense to me as a first step.

Once we returned home and John began taking melatonin, Dr. Kaufer took us through a regimen of very gradual increases, building up to 9 mg. This took a few weeks. When John's primary care doctor added another medication during this time, Dr. Kaufer stepped John back to 6 mg melatonin, so he would have time to adjust to the other new medicine. Then John resumed melatonin at 9 mg. Three years later, I found a slow release form at 10 mg, and John is using that now with doctor approval.

The process was strategic on Dr. Kaufer's part in not only letting John's body gradually adjust to a new chemical, but in doing one thing at a time. He was adamant about having only one variable to observe in order to see what would change John's symptoms for the better. The more I accepted his strategy, the calmer I became as John's symptoms slowly improved.

John's sleep, according to Dr. Kaufer's reports, went from "prominent sleep disturbance" to "still has significant residual involuntary movements" to "additional symptomatic relief, although there was still some residual 'sword fighting' movements" to "became more agitated at night" (when other medicine was introduced) to "improved sleep pattern."

All this information was conveyed using e-mails to update Dr. Kaufer while he fine-tuned the amount of melatonin until we found the level that was most effective for improving John's sleep.

Dr. Kaufer's overall approach of doing one thing at a time while giving me access to regular and clear communication with him also made me slow down and calm down in my frantic search for solutions. I was learning his style of communication, adapting to it over time, while my trust level was growing as I saw John respond well to his suggestions.

Once again, Dr. Kaufer's methods were treating me, as John's caregiver, while simultaneously treating John.

At the next appointment, with John's sleep quality improved, Dr. Kaufer prescribed the Exelon patch. It was the first day it was available for use. John responded well to it. Much later in August 2008, Namenda was added to John's regimen with a similar significant and dramatic improvement of his symptoms. He was more outgoing in social situations, more alert, more active, and cognitively brighter. His facial expression improved, and his cheeks were pink again.

By the third appointment with him, all our family members were definitely Kaufer fans. He obviously knew what he was doing.

9
Sharing Feelings with Our Son

After over a year of trying to figure out what had been happening to John while I was also managing his law office on a daily basis, I was worn out. It often had felt like I was living two lives inside of one body as I tried to cover bases for John while my own bases were being slammed on every side. I felt very traumatized at this point in the story.

Just after the first Dr. Kaufer appointment, a phone call between John David and me made it clear to him how down and depressed I was. I learned later that his response to this after hanging up was anger at me. He could not understand why I could be down after such a positive, encouraging doctor's appointment in which treatments for symptoms and a game plan was laid out to help us cope with John's LBD diagnosis. He expressed that I should be more upbeat, encouraging, and positive to help John have as many good days as possible.

From my perspective, though, Dr. Kaufer was doctor number twelve in a long, frustrating medical journey. I had had it with the medical system at this point, even as we were finally getting the answers and the help we so desperately wanted and needed. I had to have some time to process and adjust to that reality. John David did not know many of the details of what I was feeling and thinking because he was not very available during the period of seeking a diagnosis. He hated talking on the phone, which was what I needed to do to share with him.

To John David's credit, he was pretty gentle in dealing with me as I went through the emotional mine field, trying to find some peace and clarity.

Here is the e-mail exchange with my son as we struggled with the emotional impact of this disease diagnosis and caregiving realities:

Hey, JD,

I am feeling better this morning. Yesterday was rough as I was overwhelmed with emotion, but another good night's sleep and some time and TLC from loved ones has helped.

Thank you for listening and supporting. You have really given so much to make a difference, and I appreciate it. Sometimes, I know it is hard for you to understand what I am feeling and why. It has to be frustrating to you, and I never mean to diminish your own pain in dealing with what this is doing to your dad. Forgive me if I gave you that impression last night.

I think I need to try to help you see how I am feeling, and perhaps that will help you in the hard spots when I am down and depressed. Maybe I can describe it like this:

I feel like the key player in a Carolina-Duke basketball game who has been playing the whole half without a break. I have been passing the ball, catching the ball, arguing with the refs, making the baskets, missing the baskets, talking to the coach, leading the team through crunch plays, dropping the ball, bumping against the other team's players, falling down— all this with only a few chances to get a drink of water or sit down, and we are still not winning the game after all my efforts. The game won't wait for me to catch up if I am tired or need a break. I am not allowed to leave the game. I am not allowed to

drop the ball for any significant period of time. Other players may take over for short periods, but the ball will always come back to me for the overwhelming majority of the time. When other players get the ball, they usually have a teammate right beside them to help them carry the ball down the court. I don't. I carry the ball alone, except that I am often required to bounce two balls at one time while playing the game.

When I hear, "You need to be more positive," it feels like you are a fresh player coming in at the third quarter (I am not saying you just entered the game; I am saying this is how it feels.) telling me I need to ratchet up my game and do a better job. My response is likely to be to look at you in disbelief and shock and give you a response that is not satisfying to you. That is because I am very tired and still in the game with few prospects of breaks.

When I am listened to and empathized with, encouraged to hold on, even when I feel I cannot, dealt with very gently and sympathetically, I tend to bounce back quicker. It's like I need to walk through the emotions to get to the other side. My personality is basically to seek the brighter picture, and I want to continue to trust that to float to the surface.

And it may be that for a couple of days after some doctor visits, I may hit these low points and need some extra TLC or just to be alone or maybe to be with someone who can just love me through it and help me to crystallize my thoughts and feelings.

For right now, I have a short-term plan:

- *Finish paperwork at office*
- *Move office furniture and equipment to the house and figure out where to put it*
- *Take a couple of days at the lake while John stays with Paige*
- *Set up computer stuff from office at house*

- *Figure out how to do taxes*
- *Buy new grill*
- *Set up regular recipes/menus for improved diet in more systematic way*

I love you! Thank you again for all you are doing. It is good to have you there. For example, by coming to the house and looking at the headphones, you enabled your dad to enjoy using them—he is in there right now listening to Shawshank while he treads away!

Take care and much love,
Mom

John David responded:

Mom,

Thank you for the e-mail and I'm glad you're feeling better. I was really thrown off last night when we talked and I found you depressed since I expected that you'd come out of such a wonderful diagnosis for Dad, full of hope, options, and promise.

You've done a fabulous job with researching, fighting through the health care system, and ensuring that Dad has great care. It's been a really long slog. I understand this, and I think you should take some time and take care of yourself. I like your plan of action.

It seems like you've gotten Dad to a much better place now, and every month since January he's been improving dramatically. I hope this will bring you some relief and comfort. You've clearly got him on the right path, and Dr. Kaufer's visit confirmed that for me loud and clear. GREAT JOB!

I love you,
JD

When I read that e-mail over again, what sticks out to me is the use of the term "wonderful diagnosis" by our son, John David. If you are a caregiver of a loved one with LBD, I am sure you would never use those two words together. I think my son was referring to the hope that Dr. Kaufer offered in terms of treatment options and the prospect of having more good times together as a family before the onset of later stages of LBD.

But John David's comment about "wonderful diagnosis" points to another element that has been a recurring theme in our relationship. It speaks to what I think is a disconnection that he has with what is really going on daily in this disease and the caregiving part that I must play. He refuses to call frequently or hesitates to stay on the phone for an extended time when I finally give up waiting for him to call and telephone him. This puts him in a position of not hearing details that are keys to understanding some things that are happening or the level of their impact on me and his dad. He assumes that he knows much more than he really knows. He assumes that he can surmise the whole truth from the small bits of information that I have shared, that Paige has shared with him, or that he has witnessed for himself.

John David comments that "I was really thrown off last night when we talked and I found you depressed…" That reveals a significant void of information and understanding that had preceded the first Dr. Kaufer appointment. His sister, Paige, had no problem understanding my depression because she had been privy to so much more information in talking with me in the months prior to the appointment.

This issue is still present in our relationship to some degree. However, when John David read the first draft of this book, he seemed to gain more insight and empathy, which is a good thing. He admitted that he learned things he had not known before. It is probably one of my best reasons for writing the book. Our son will graciously take the time to sit down to read and edit my account on paper, though he still struggles to receive it in the smaller daily unfolding of the story.

Different members of our family have responded in a variety of ways to John's diagnosis and its aftermath. Some have drawn closer; others have backed away somewhat. The disease has an impact on everyone in one way or another. Thankfully, both our children have been there for us in different ways that reflect who they are.

10
Office Building is Sold

In the middle of everything else that was going on, the office had to be closed down, with appropriate storage of files and handling of all the financial matters. The biggest financial matter initially was selling the building where the law practice had been. All that fell to me.

I designed a leaflet and did some small advertising. When we would get a call, I would show it and give its background and history. It helped me to explain how it had been used over the years, its unique features, and how much we had enjoyed our ten years there. Even though there was some stress involved, it kept me busy, and I think that helped me during the first few months after we retired.

Once a local young attorney realized our building was on the market, he made offers, we negotiated, and it was sold to him. A big stressor was removed from my plate, and there was more in the retirement portfolio to boot. This was one area where we felt totally good that our efforts had produced a favorable outcome with no downside. It gave John and me a boost.

11
Ongoing House Search Ends

After the diagnosis and meltdown at Paige's house, I still spent hours on real estate Web sites, hours driving around looking at neighborhoods near my children's homes with enough distance to address Dave's concern of being too close. The urge to move was powerful. When Doctor Number Eleven stressed how we needed to settle near our children and prepare for the worst, my fear of being alone fighting this monster increased, and fear is a powerful motivator.

I set up an appointment at a pretty retirement residence/ assisted living place in Chapel Hill. When the materials arrived, I read the prices and saw what you received for your money. I realized it was more than we wanted to spend on that option, so I cancelled the appointment. That option had much less to offer than what we were enjoying in our own beautiful home at this stage.

The search for homes in the triangle area went on for months. Finally, John and I decided that our best choice was to stay where we were. Over time with Paige's, my friend Glenda's, and my mother's daily supportive calls, frequent visits back and forth to enjoy our grandson, and loving support from other friends in Rutherford County, my mind and emotions slowed down. There was an easing of the frantic scrambling for a new place to be, and I was able to see the good things we already had.

Our house is elder friendly with wide doorways, large rooms, and a first-floor master bedroom suite. Even our stairs are designed to be relatively easy to move up and down. Our large screened porch comes with a pretty view, and twice a day church bells chime hymns softly through the trees. With some key remodeling, we felt we could make this place work for us for quite a while.

We had good friends in this small town where we had put down roots thirty years earlier. My close friend, Glenda Jowers, was more like a sister and touched base with us every day. For three decades, she had been a consistent and sweet confidante who would be impossible to replace. If we needed to move later, we would cross that bridge when we came to it. In the meantime, I would drive a lot to see our grandson and other grandchildren as they began to arrive.

We also thought this place would make a good grandchild haven for spending time with them. John loved his yard and garden areas where he could putter as he wished.

One fall weekend our children visited with the goal of developing a more convenient garden spot for John. They also planted plum trees by the driveway, and we enhanced the strawberry patch in the backyard.

Over time we had a small side porch and sloping sidewalk added to allow entry to the house with no steps. We remodeled the downstairs bathroom and made it handicap friendly. Both changes, which I describe in more detail later in the book, added beauty and value to our home and made us happier with our decision to stay.

12

Still Emotionally Fragile

By February 2008, eight months had passed since John's diagnosis by Doctor Number Eleven. I was still not myself. I decided to reach out to someone who might be able to give me some hope about getting back to feeling normal again. This was the e-mail I sent to the Lewy Body Dementia Association Web site help-line coordinator.

Can someone tell me how long is the "normal" adjustment period after finding out my husband's diagnosis of this nightmare? Should I expect to feel this emotionally fragile from now on? The least thing or criticism can send me into a downward emotional spiral when I am used to being a very strong person.

The LBDA Help-line Coordinator answered me. She expressed sympathy for my situation and feelings and shared that her husband also had LBD. In response to my question, she said that her best answer is "until you adjust." She was gentle and kind, but basically said that you could not put a time frame on it. She also encouraged me to join a spouse caregiver group and to take care of my own health.

I had tried going on the LBDA Web site discussion forum after John's diagnosis in June 2007 and found myself getting more depressed and worried when I read about some of the struggles that caregivers were having with loved ones farther into the disease than John. It was not very productive for me at that time.

I needed to just cope with each day and find my bearings without a lot of "what ifs" to consider. I still have mixed feelings about reading the struggles of others because this disease varies with each person. What one patient does may never happen to another. The last thing I wanted to do was borrow trouble that may never come our way.

I checked in to the Web site now and again to keep up with the latest developments in research, but I had to limit myself at this early stage to not dwelling on what might happen in the future.

It is important here to make clear that there can be wonderful reassurance from talking with other caregivers. I have seen posts on the discussion forums where a specific problem was responded to by multiple caregivers with good potential solutions. It helps to have someone who is on a similar journey as your own to share your heart with. That is very valuable. Hopefully, one day there will be a place in online discussion forums for early stage LBD caregivers to share and encourage one another.

13
Jason is Born

Sometimes you get a broadside hit unexpectedly when you are in the position of caregiver of a disease like LBD. The birth of our second grandchild, Jason, was one of those times for me.

On September 24, 2008, everything was going well in the Caesarean birth process. Jason was born healthy, and Dave invited us see him in the nursery as nurses were cleaning and swaddling him. I was so excited to look for the first time at this precious new person in our lives. Being a Nana has been one of the most amazing joys of my life. When we arrived at the nursery, I noticed that John went and sat in a nearby chair, reading a magazine instead of looking through the window at Jason. That bothered me. John had always made his family connections a high priority in his life, so this was just not like him.

Here was a huge family event, but he had focused on some prints on the wall as we had walked to the nursery area. His attention was not on the baby at all. He finally got out of the chair and looked briefly inside the window at Jason, but returned to reading his magazine. I can remember looking at him in that chair and thinking, "How can you just sit there when this new little grandchild has just arrived? I want you to come over here and stand with me and look at this precious child."

Sometimes LBD does this kind of thing. The person with it is socially and emotionally removed from what is going on.

A couple of hours later while eating lunch with my mother, a wave of depression came over me. I just sank into sadness. I stayed there for several weeks, mourning what John and I would lose as grandparents together with all our grandchildren. I had to let go of that dream, and over time, I allowed myself to do that.

I believe the process of allowing yourself to let go of former dreams can make room for the new possibilities. I could create a new way of grandparenting that was still joyful, and that was what I tried to do. Being the best possible Nana for my grandchildren is fabulous medicine. Time spent with them reenergizes my spirit.

I focused on being a fun Nana. I sang to them with gusto, visited them often, cuddled with deep appreciation for each embrace, and called my grandsons for personal conversations as soon as they could even say my name. My children and I use video telephoning. If John wants to join in, he is encouraged to do so, but I stopped letting myself focus on what he would not or could not do. I just enjoy the moments when he chooses to be engaged while I stay engaged myself.

I still sometimes mourn what might have been for us as grandparents—like taking them on trips together to see our wonderful country. But I try to focus on what we can do and accentuate the positive moments and memories. I refuse to let LBD rob me or my grandchildren of sweet moments and memories.

14

A Letter to Dr. Number Eleven

John had made progress since July 2007, when he first saw Dr. Kaufer at UNC. In the year and a half since then, he had returned to us emotionally and socially as a result of the therapies prescribed by Dr. Kaufer and all the efforts of family members and friends to keep both of us supported so well. By this time John's sleep quality had improved with the use of melatonin. His conversation, sense of humor, and social connectedness had improved with the use of the Exelon patch and Namenda. I had become calmer inside and able to live more in the moment.

However, I had a simmering issue with the neurologist who had sent John and my daughter on their way after a devastating diagnosis of LBD, with its horrifying definition, but with minimal options to provide help. That neurologist, whom I call Dr. Number Eleven, recommended good nutrition and exercise routines and advice to find a place to live where John could easily transition into a nursing home. He had advised getting financial matters in order and preparing for the end but had refused to provide any medications to help with symptom relief. Even the next visit was to be with his nurse practitioner and not with him. John left this guy's exam room with no hope at all.

The lack of hope from this doctor was later confirmed when I sent him a barrage of e-mail questions, which he graciously answered. Dr. Number Eleven made it clear in his response to my question about medicines that might help John with some of his symptoms that he was not inclined to offer that option to John and that it might even be dangerous to do so.

After seeing the radically different approach by Dr. Kaufer and living with its wonderful impact on John and the rest of the family, I was ready to let Dr. Number Eleven know two things: his impact on John and his opportunity to offer better options to his current patients.

I could not help but think of how Dr. Number Eleven's patients were settling for what he had to offer and how they might be sinking into a black hole of hopelessness if they took his option as the only way to approach this disease, especially in the early stages.

So at the end of 2008, I sat down at my computer and, using his real name, sent Dr. Number Eleven this e-mail.

Dear "Dr. Number Eleven,"

My husband was diagnosed by you in June 2007, with LBD. He was sent home with suggestions for diet and exercise and told he would see one of your staff members at his next visit. John told me he left your office with no hope.

*I did some research and made an appointment with Dr. Dan Kaufer at UNC to verify your diagnosis and see if more proactive treatment might be available to help us with daily life. John is thriving under Dr. Kaufer's care of **aggressive treatment of symptoms as early as possible**. He and his staff have told us that they have numerous patients who are doing well after five to six years of this approach to LBD.*

We understand that LBD is a progressive disease, but we were told at UNC that, like other conditions, there are many treatments to help alleviate symptoms. We appreciate the

compassion and understanding of this treatment plan, which
preserves personhood at optimal levels as long as possible.

John left Dr. Kaufer's office the first time with hope. He sees Dr. Kaufer every six months and continues to enjoy daily life so much more fully now, and his whole family can see a big difference in him due to this treatment plan.

Please consider it for your other patients with LBD.

Dr. Number Eleven replied the next day. He thanked me for my "thoughtful letter," said he was glad we had found Dr. Kaufer, describing him as skilled and caring, and then said he would consider my suggestions carefully.

I was pleased with his response and hoped that he would begin to offer more aggressive treatment of symptoms to his patients with LBD. However, in late 2011, I met another caregiver wife whose husband was also diagnosed with LBD by Dr. Number Eleven in 2007. As I talked with her, I learned that this doctor had not changed his treatment strategy for LBD patients much after all. Her husband had not done well under his care. She had trusted that a reputable doctor at a reputable hospital would do the right things, but in 2011, she decided to flee from this kind of approach to LBD.

When this diagnosis hits you and your family, it is overwhelming. You desperately want to find some answer somewhere that will make things better, even if for a short while. You want the time with your loved one to be quality time. You need hope and options, not defeat and resignation.

My point in sharing this information is that as a patient or caregiver, you do not have to remain silent in dealing with doctors. They are human beings with flaws and limitations, and they have various abilities and sensitivities in dealing with others. They and their future patients can benefit from feedback and new information from their current or past patients.

Some need to be reminded that they are working every day with flesh and blood people who have hearts that are breaking and who need hope as much as they need scientific expertise. When a doctor is as far off base as I believe Dr. Number Eleven was, it may help another person in a similar situation to your own if you take the time to let that doctor know he may need to reconsider what he is doing to his patients by the choices he has made.

Doctors need to get this. Even if they cannot cure the disease, they can help tremendously by alleviating some of the symptoms, if only for a season. And hope is some of the best medicine of all.

15
Build a Ramp

At this point in the spring of 2009, John and I both felt good about staying in our house even though we lived over two hundred miles from our children and grandchildren. We decided to work with the good features of our home that already made it senior friendly.

An obstacle for us when John was diagnosed was the primary entry to our home. There were two steps that were uneven and the storm door was ultra heavy, so that when you came and went, you felt off balance. I knew that if we upgraded this entrance attractively while taking care of John's need for a smooth steady walk into the house, we could have a good investment all around.

Taking this on as a creative challenge turned a taxing renovation experience into a more positive one. It made me feel more in control of what was happening. I thought of the money used to change our house as funds I would have given to a nursing home earlier than necessary, if I did not invest it now. I also viewed it as a way to beautify our home to make it more marketable in case we needed to sell and move closer to family.

After months of thinking about what to do to improve the situation, I was speaking with a contractor about putting up a small deck type of porch with a ramp-style exit to the driveway. He suggested a cement ramp with a semicircle-shaped porch combination that could be stamped to give it a slate look, and I immediately knew that was the answer. It would be safe, easy to use, and attractive with flowers added on each side.

I ended up drawing the picture of what I wanted and expanding on the original concept. The entry today is prettier than my front entrance and a delight to use as we pack the car to go see grandkids or bring in the groceries.

A problem was turned into a plus. It was money well spent. The cost was about one-fourth of one month's nursing home bill in our community. I would much rather invest our money in home improvement than in nursing home care.

This project is an example of turning lemons that life may give you into lemonade. Almost every time we walk in or out of our pretty entry way, we smile at the transformation. It is one of our little treasures we get to enjoy on a daily basis.

16
A Bathroom That Works

One of the smartest choices I have made in caregiving was the early remodeling of the bathroom. My caregiving friends all told me the bathroom was a crucial point of stress for them. Once again I was choosing to invest in home improvement proactively to postpone the need for possible earlier nursing home support.

We had a traditional bathroom with a combination tub/shower and floor-mounted toilet that was not going to work with movement issues for John or for me as I aged with back problems.

I decided to gut the old bathroom and start from scratch in order to get what we needed. LBD presented two major problems in the bathroom—how to bathe if a walker or wheelchair was in our future and how to deal with inevitable messes around the toilet.

The key to solving both these issues was to use the back half of our bathroom as a "wet zone" and remove all obstacles to cleaning and stepping into the bath area. I designed a tile floor that gently sloped toward a single drain in the shower area, using a European model of shower design. It is also like an American commercial bathroom floor.

Floor tiles are the one-inch size, so the floor is not slippery. There is no raised lip that separates the shower from the rest of the bathroom. Instead, the back half of our bathroom floor gently slopes toward the drain from any point, so that any water on the floor moves into the drain. This also makes it easy to bring in a shower chair when it is needed—there are no barriers on the floor and there is the feeling of having a lot more space. The caregiver can easily maneuver all around the chair in this setting to help with bathing. The showerhead faces toward the wet zone and away from the dry zone of the whole room.

The toilet, which is placed in the "wet zone," is a wall hung type by American Standard, so that cleaning under it is a matter of reaching for the handheld showerhead with a seven-foot hose, turning on the hottest water to rinse the floor and the undersides of the toilet, spraying antibacterial cleaner, and rinsing everything into the drain at that end of the bathroom. Let the hot water, the floor design, and the cleanser do the work for you. There is no getting on the hands and knees to scrub around the base of a toilet involved, so stress levels and back issues stay low.

I selected attractive oval-shaped handholds for the shower and toilet areas. They do the job with a sense of style. Another addition was a motion-sensitive overhead light, which turns on automatically when you step in or near the bathroom door.

Besides these upgrades, the other item that has been a blessing to us is the toilet bidet seat. It is an expensive item, but has been worth it. We chose the top-of-the line bidet seat by Toto that has a remote that I mounted onto the wall next to the toilet with heavy-duty Velcro.

A bidet seat acts like a bidet, in that it washes you after going to the bathroom, but it takes the place of a normal toilet seat on top of a regular toilet. This is helpful for back issues and any movement problems because the work is done mostly by the seat's cleaning sprays, and all you have to do is dry yourself with a few sheets of toilet paper without the usual twisting and turning needed with regular toilet cleaning.

After we started to use the bidet seat, we realized that it also helps with issues of constipation because the warm sprays actually help to relax that part of the body to make going to the bathroom easier. My husband, who was a skeptic, is now a believer in bidet seats. For me as a caregiver, this will help in the future when assisting John with cleaning will be more of an issue. I think that this item alone can keep John at home for extra months because it reduces both the stress and some of the physical labor involved with toileting.

Not long after remodeling, the new bathroom was put to the test when the toilet overflowed. What would have taken two hours to clean with significant back stress took me about twenty minutes with no back stress. It was not hard or stressful thanks to the new room design. Both of us were glad that we had changed the space to be more user-friendly, sooner rather than later.

17
Little Reminders

In February 2009, I had been away for a few days visiting grandchildren in the Triangle area of the state. John had stayed at home alone. Grandbaby Nate had been born to Liz and John David a few weeks earlier, and this was a happy time in the family. Our children and grandchildren were all thriving and doing well. There was much to be thankful for.

As I chatted on the phone, I was cleaning up the kitchen counter. I noticed a large red stain on the countertop close to the sink.

"I wonder what happened here while I was gone," I said.

Then I opened the refrigerator door, and there was a splatter of red on the center shelf that had congealed and dripped down the edge onto the lower section.

"Hmmm. It is always interesting to come back and find proof that some mysterious event occurred and left a little evidence behind."

This kind of thing happens with almost every short-term visit I make away from home these days. These little reminders often feed a level of quiet stress—an awareness that all is not well underneath the veneer of calm that I work so hard to maintain in our home.

Another time, I walked into the kitchen and found five cabinet doors gaping open. I thought, "John must have emptied the dishwasher," as I closed each door. It had happened twice before that week.

For what feels like the thousandth time on another day, there is a full tilt search for John's glasses. Thinking I would solve things, I bought three pairs of reading glasses for him to have a set by the bed, by his favorite chair, and one hidden away. On this hunt all three pairs seem to have vanished into thin air.

Getting dressed some days can be a challenge. How he can manage to twist a shirt into the confused tangle that it becomes is beyond me. We often just laugh about it to relieve the tension. Then he may ask me to put on one of his socks for him.

Over and over again, John has to be reminded to comb his hair, take a bath, brush his teeth, and shave. He seems content to sit in his recliner for days while considering none of the above as worth his time and energy.

18
Old Wounds

After one of my trips away from home, I returned to find something that broke my heart. It did not have anything to do with LBD. John just left something around that he had intended to hide.

It brought up old wounds from the past. I confronted him about it and let him know this was a deal breaker for me unless he was ready to deal with his issues. He agreed to do whatever I wanted to work on the problem.

I am not comfortable going into detail about the particulars here, but I feel it is important to share that old wounds of any sort can rear up at tough times in your journey as a married couple. When you are dealing with a monster like LBD, it can feel hugely overwhelming.

I got in touch with a counselor, who was part of an out-of-state organization we had supported. She gave me some good advice and direction for dealing with the issue in conjunction with LBD. This counselor said that John might be helped with some aspects of the LBD by effective counseling. I did not understand that at all, but it sounded good. John and I planned to travel across the country to have intensive counseling to help us.

But the more I thought about it, the more I became concerned about what the stress of the long trip and the intensive nature of the counseling might do to John's health on a permanent basis. We opted to try to get an appointment locally with a counselor we had visited briefly years before. That was one of the wisest decisions of our lives.

Most relationships have some history and some issues that are unresolved. These issues tend to become more exaggerated in the process of struggling with a new diagnosis as well as coping with long-term caregiving of a loved one. What the disease brings all by itself in terms of frustrating symptoms and fears is significant.

I have found that counseling has been tremendously helpful both for me and for John. We have learned how to communicate better so that each of us is actually hearing and appreciating what is being said by the other. We also now understand much better those things that are most important to the other and those things that trigger stress. This is invaluable in improving the quality of our daily lives.

John said that our psychologist, Dr. Terry Ledford, has contributed in some ways as much to his feeling of well-being as has his neurologist and the medicines he has prescribed. I asked him to elaborate on that. John said that he has a clearer understanding of his feelings and of my feelings and knows better how to cope with things as a result of the counseling.

"It has given greater clarity to me," he said.

19
Love Makes a Big Difference

John and I sat in comfortable chairs in Dr. Terry Ledford's office in January 2010. He was a psychologist whom we both trusted and who had helped us wrestle with this monster called LBD for a year at this point. He also was helping us with more effective communication. At our first visit, I had emphasized to him that we needed to control stress as we dealt with tough issues, because stress can make LBD much worse quickly.

I told him that I had laughed out loud many times since last week when I had asked him with my heart on my sleeve, "Do you think he really loves me?"

He had assured me that John really did love me by saying, "Are you crazy? Of course, he loves you! It is so obvious."

I thought it was hilarious that a psychologist was asking me if I was crazy. But his words have provided an anchor that I would not trade for the entire world.

They told me that John's love for me was real and had been there all along, even when I could not see it or feel it, because John is one of those quiet guys who think you should just know it without having to hear it. This is so unbelievably important. That sure knowledge of his love for me will be a storehouse I may need to draw from someday when John cannot actually say the words that I want and need to hear.

On this visit, the issue was letting John know that when he chooses to dress too casually or to go out in public with food stains on his shirt, that it creates fear in me. The fear comes from how it makes him look. All John had to do was to dress with a collared shirt, long dark pants, and to be clean with combed hair. Then he presents an image in public that reflects that he is a retired professional. It maintains a place of more peace and security for us both. When he looked bad, he looked sicker.

I was finally able to deeply feel what I was trying to say while I was saying it, not to just intellectualize it. I was able to express it in such a way that John could better hear my fears. There were tears in my eyes as I spoke to him.

Dr. Ledford supported and underlined what I said and affirmed the validity of my concerns. He helped John see not only that my position was reasonable and valid emotionally, but that John had earned the right to present himself as a retired professional in public with the benefits that come with that. John's expression changed, and he seemed to really "get it" at last.

I was so grateful that Dr. Ledford backed me up so affectively and effectively.

Then Dr. Ledford helped me to see that by communicating my concerns to John in a softer way, by sharing my fears and hurts as the basis for my request for a change in his actions, that John was able to hear what I was saying better and did not feel criticized by my words. When I spoke in frustration, anger, or irritation, the deeper feelings were missed, and the problem did not get solved. I needed to practice this more.

Because I was a more extroverted and outspoken, strong woman, and John was more quiet and easy going, I knew that I needed to develop some specific ways to talk to him when he needs to be motivated to get up out of the recliner and turn off the TV.

I was presented with a dilemma when the neurologist and the counselor gave what appeared to be conflicting directions to me. The neurologist said at our last appointment, "Be a drill sergeant. No guilt. Do what you have to do to get him moving. He will lose it if he does not use it."

But the counselor had said, "Be soft in your words. Be vulnerable." So how was I to pull off both at the same time?

I asked Dr. Ledford for some specific words to say to John to help me with this. He gave me these ways to soften my words when I see John getting into an introverted rut:

"Let's go for a ride" (when John is too passive or watching too much TV).

"I'm probably being a little crazy here, but..."

"I may be worrying too much here, but..."

"I know I'm being the drill sergeant here, but..."

"I don't want you to feel criticized or pushed, so let me know if I make you feel that way."

This way I am addressing the problem with a softer, but firm approach to get John to do what will help him to stay more active. It feels like a good example of loving him.

I have also become bolder about expressing exactly what I want emotionally from John. If I need to be held or told that I am loved, I make that plain and clear. John has learned over time with the help of our counselor to respond well to that. He uses more words and more often expresses what he is thinking and feeling.

As a result we both feel more loved by the other. This shift in communication styles has created more happiness for both of us.

20
Just Say It

In a March 2010 counseling session, Dr. Ledford did a very simple thing—it may even sound silly at first. He told John to just look into my eyes and say, "I really love you."

I got a big lump in my throat as soon as he said it. This was huge for me, hearing what I wanted so much to hear from John, who is one of those guys who just takes it for granted that you know.

At first John's attempt was a little awkward. He said, "I love you," while looking in my direction.

Terry said, "Look in her eyes and say, 'I *really* love you.'"

Then John one-upped him. He looked into my eyes and said, "I really love you, Patsy Anne."

I melted.

"Say it again," I said. He did.

Waves of relief and love washed over me. I could feel a soft healing and a recharging taking place inside.

Then Terry told John to do that every day and whenever I asked him to do it at home or wherever we were. He has complied and even initiated it some on his own.

My response has been clear and positive, and he seems encouraged to keep doing it. The difference it is making is dramatic and very good. Knowing that I am deeply loved by him makes things so much easier.

Shortly after we returned home, John was doing a favor for me and commented, "I am doing this because I love you." The goodness of the feeling that washed over me in that moment was actually physical—my shoulders relaxed, I took a deep breath to expand the sweet presence of that love. I felt like I would go to the moon and back for him if he asked me.

At moments like this, the choice of counseling as a caregiver option seems wise indeed. It is likely that without counseling we would never have learned how to communicate with each other in as meaningful a way as we do now. I could have died never knowing for sure how much John loved me and never being able to tell him how much I loved him in ways that would penetrate to his core. There is a level of peace, deep joy, and gratitude that John and I now enjoy as a result.

21
Stay in the Moment

In March 2010, I was e-mailing Jean, a friend who was a former paralegal in John's law practice. I told her that John and I missed what had felt like a good team ministry in which we tried to help people. I said to her, "But life has different chapters for God's different purposes."

It is hard for me to imagine how anyone gets through such a hard place in life as an LBD diagnosis of one's spouse without a strong faith. I am a believer in Jesus Christ. That belief and what comes with it has been a source of tremendous strength and grace in this journey. It has given me unconditional love and unexplainable energy.

My faith has allowed me to focus my energy and effort. Instead of dwelling on the inevitable "Why?", I have been able to move on to the more productive question of "What are You up to, Lord?" Other ways of saying this are "What are You teaching us? Where do we grow in this? What are the lessons we are supposed to learn on this part of our life journey with You?"

When the questions change, the answers present themselves more clearly.

After the early traumatic months of adjusting to this new season of our lives, John and I settled down in our lovely home. We dwelled on our blessings, our family, our friends, and each other. We made the conscious decision to live in each day as fully as we could, but with a laid back focus of "stopping to smell the roses along the way." We made sitting on the porch together and listening to the birds sing a full event unto itself. We commented often about how our home with its pretty pastoral view provided a kind of vacation spot for us. Both of us determined to look for the good. We found it, and it was and is sweet.

Our faith reinforced our decisions. It is full of hope and promises, and we opted to claim both.

I surrounded myself with close friends who are like-minded folks. They are people who believe in the power of prayer and the strength that faith provides for difficult times. I contact them often, some of them even daily, to share our lives and to be encouraged to hold fast to God when the going gets a bit rough. From what they tell me, I have encouraged them as well with some of my choices in this journey.

The Bible has been a source of strength, and hymns and songs of praise have lifted our spirits on many a day. John loves to hear me sing. Sometimes our long car rides to visit grandchildren include songs of praise as we roll down the highway. It is free and brings smiles to both of us. Our batteries feel recharged after a couple of songs just praising God.

We also share *Kid's Praise* CDs with our grandchildren. As we listen with them, we are uplifted. It also gives us a chance to share our faith with them as they grow and learn about God.

Quiet Bible study can be like food and nourishment at a time like this. Just what is needed for that day often presents itself. It feels like you line yourself up with God in that day's part of the journey. The essence of what you read may get passed along later in a phone call with a friend. Direction for a better way to handle a small crisis may come clearly in those quiet study times.

growing in this chapter of my life journey—even if it
es painful. The biggest lesson for me is to stay in each
nd each day, lining up with God for that time. When
I can stay in the moment and be open to learning what God has
for me and for us, then great peace and even joy are in that day.

I can feel myself getting softer, calmer, gentler, and more
empathetic.

Staying in the moment has also been a cornerstone of what
our counselor, Dr. Terry Ledford, has encouraged John and me
to do. Many times he has reminded us, "You cannot change
what happened yesterday. Your fears for tomorrow may never
materialize. But you live in this moment. You can choose how to
do that because it is real. Yesterday and tomorrow exist only in
your mind."

This act of living fully in the moment is a working out of my
faith and trust in God to give John and me what we need each
day. Jesus taught this when he said in the last two verses of the
sixth chapter of the Gospel of Matthew, "Seek first the kingdom
of God and His righteousness, and all these things shall be added
unto you. Therefore, do not worry about tomorrow, for tomorrow
will worry about itself."

22
A Trip to the Keys

John and I hunkered down and put off travel, except to visit family, for almost three years. Travel had been our hobby and had brought us so many wonderful experiences and memories. But I think we were afraid to try it in case it made him worse. Or maybe I just needed to get some balance and calm back into my life.

When we asked his neurologist about traveling to Europe about a year after we met him, he said we might try it, but that there was some risk involved. Stress can make LBD patients get worse pretty quickly, so we decided against that trip.

Around Christmas of 2009 we started to plan a vacation trip to the Florida Keys. There were some components for any travel plans that I felt were important for keeping John stable, calm, and healthy.

I wanted to choose a nonstop flight to minimize airport travel issues, and I wanted to settle into no more than two spots as our home bases while there. Activities needed to take into account John's lack of stamina and issues with movement.

In April 2010, we arrived at the airport to fly to Florida for a week in the Keys. Inside the airport John sat in a wheelchair for the first time as I pushed him from spot to spot so that we could move quickly and smoothly with no stress on him. That was emotional for me, but it also put us in the front of every line, which was helpful. John seemed to be fine with it.

We landed in Miami and rented a Mustang convertible as a happy nod to the car in which we began dating. As we pulled out of the airport car rental terminal, I raised my arms and shouted a loud cheer into the sunny, beautiful afternoon. We were young and moving again with the wind in our hair. John laughed.

Nice rooms in quality resorts gave us the security of safe and pleasant accommodations. When we arrived, I spoke to the folks at the front desk, explaining that we had received a bad diagnosis and that this was likely our last vacation together. We were given great upgrades in both places on the spot.

John had always done the planning for our many past vacations. This time, I did it, but not by choice. At our two destinations, I had planned for us to do things that would not be too physically demanding on John. We were able to tour on a glass-bottomed boat and view the seabed miles away from shore. We took an exciting ride in the Everglades with alligators all around us, sitting right up front where we would get wet as we did 360s in the grassy wetlands. There was a small but nice bird sanctuary near our first resort hotel in Key Largo where we took our time walking through the pathway to the Gulf. Just driving around and looking at the changing colors of the water and the sunsets was relaxing.

At Hawks Cay, the second resort, John tended to stay inside the plush townhouse while I went to the pool. That was poignant for me. It felt lonely, but he was happy to be in such a lovely place and looked forward to the good meals and drives we enjoyed together. So the trip was bittersweet, and our activities were low-key and more laid back than they would have been before he was sick. I did include one of my "Life List" goals. I swam with the dolphins while we were there. John watched from the viewing balcony, though he wilted some in the sun as I romped in the water. But it was a good decision to do something special just for myself.

We may take another big trip, and we may not. Fortunately we live in a beautiful part of the country where it is easy to take short road trips and see the lovely North Carolina mountains or beaches. There is something to be said for a day of drinking in the local color and sleeping in your own bed that night.

23
Revisiting Our Life Together

I stayed up late to watch two chick flicks while John had already gone to bed. There was a scene in one of the movies where a couple is in Europe sitting beside a large pool with fountains. It took me back to a scene from my own past that was a highlight in our lives.

It was the summer of 2002. John and I were in Tuscany at a wonderful hotel that had a huge pool with fountains on each edge. The water would arch over to the other side when the fountains were turned on. We were sitting poolside, enjoying finger foods and a wonderful bottle of wine we had bought that day in a little Tuscan village. This was where John asked me if I would be interested in coming to work for him in his law office. I could not believe my ears. What an intriguing idea! We sat for a long time as the sun set beautifully over the Tuscan hills, and we talked about what it might be like to work together. A big part of it could be arranging our schedules to be able to take more vacations like this.

Now I look back on this memory and am so glad and grateful that we had the opportunity to travel and share great places with each other. We did it early instead of waiting until retirement. If we had waited, we would have lost the chance to live that dream together.

After the movie ended, I went upstairs and snuggled up next to John and told him about seeing the fountain. We spent a few minutes reliving that wonderful time in Tuscany. I cried and told him I never wanted to be without him. He cried, too. But it was a sweet time together remembering and holding one another. We both cherish these times when we can revisit our lives as a couple.

It is important to take advantage of times like this when a memory pops into your mind. You should stop what you are doing and relive it with your loved one.

It can be as simple as going through a photo album together or listening to a favorite old song. LBD slows down everything, so why not use that opportunity to walk down memory lane in the early stage? It will enrich that day, and it will enrich your heart.

24

To Dream the Impossible Dream

I read some of Ginnie Burkholder's eloquent essays on the LBDA Web site. She spoke of her husband being her Don Quixote, which resonated with me. John has always seen himself that way. It is probably one of the reasons I love him so much. He has always been idealistic and has wanted to make a difference, especially for people who have no connections, no clout in this world. He played that out so many times in his work as an attorney and a prosecutor.

The song that we both loved when we began dating was "The Impossible Dream." I would sometimes sing it to him as we drove around together and we would talk about our dreams.

It hit me earlier today that I, like so many other caregivers, am living out the lyrics of this song.

Now I have taken up John's mantle. Now I am the Don Quixote. Now I dream an impossible dream that this monster disease will go away. I fight an unbeatable, progressive, relentless foe. I bear with sometimes unbearable sorrow, and I daily walk where many a brave person would dare not go if given a choice.

There are many like me. Maybe you are one of them. When others do not understand us and what we are going through, it helps to remember that. We are not alone.

25
Change of Focus on Book

In October 2010, my daughter and I were talking about how I was changing the target of my writings to early stage caregiving, because I could not find any books that addressed those issues in any depth. She was encouraging me and affirming that decision.

She said, "Mom, what if you had not persisted and just stayed with that first neurologist, who gave us no sense of hope at all? Think of where Pops might be today. Other people need to know how important it is to keep looking until you get the right doctor. And that is just one of the things you did to make it better for Pops."

My eyes filled with tears at her words.

Comments like that make me determined to get the word out that things can be done to make it better, at least for a while. And this is what matters. We cannot cheat death, but to postpone the inevitable is to get more meaningful days.

26
You Were Always on My Mind

In late October 2010, my mother came for a few days to visit and enjoy the beautiful fall leaves in the North Carolina mountains not far from our home. John rode in the backseat with us as we climbed into the colors and put on some music that all of us would enjoy as we traveled.

The CD that everyone wanted to hear was by Willie Nelson, one with his best hits. We were all into the music as the fall panorama unfolded before us, and then song number seven came on—"You Were Always on My Mind."

As the words poured out of the speakers, I got a lump in my throat. My eyes moved to the rearview mirror, and there were John's eyes looking into mine. We held each other's gaze. It was one of those moments when nothing is said and everything is said in the absence of words.

Getting through the entire song in silence without bursting into tears as I was driving along with my mother there in the front seat was a challenge. The words of the song spoke our love story, here in the later chapters of our lives, but we could not talk about it then.

Later I took my mother home and visited with the grandchildren for a few days. Those were sweet days with sweet memories. John stayed home, and we both got a little break from our routine.

On my way home, the first day of November, I decided to play Willie Nelson songs again. This time I was alone in the car, driving down I-85, sobbing my heart out, as Willie crooned those poignant lyrics.

I called John and said, "When I get home I want to put on 'You Were Always on My Mind.' I want you to dance with me to that song over and over again until I say that is enough."

John agreed immediately. When I arrived in the driveway at home, he met me at the door, hugged me, and said, "Where is the Willie Nelson CD?"

We put it on and danced in the middle of the kitchen until I could stop crying. He held me and kissed my cheek so sweetly. I could feel the gentle, deep love from him at long last.

It was one of the most moving and healing moments of my marriage to John. It was a treasure in the darkness.

27
I Yam What I Yam

John and I had a 9:00 a.m. appointment in November 2010, with Dr. Terry Ledford, our counselor. I somehow forgot that morning. The office had called, asking where we were, which was embarrassing and upsetting. Dr. Ledford is in great demand, and it is hard to get another appointment on short notice. We were going to have to wait another month to see him, which was not good. However, his office called right back, saying that the person with the 10:00 a.m. appointment had arrived early. So we could have that time if we could be there by ten.

"Great!" I said.

I was off to the races, zipping around, jumping up to prepare to take my shower and get dressed. We had been lounging around over coffee up to that point.

John's reaction was different. "Next time I don't want you to make an appointment on such short notice. This is too much."

The feeling of having to rush to get ready was upsetting to him. Fortunately, I was able to step back and see that right away. In the past, I would have let him know that I disagreed with him, but this time I handled it differently.

I said, "John, there is no pressure here, no rushing needed. All you have to do is shower, shave, and dress. Shaving is optional if it causes you too much stress."

While I was saying this, I was laying out his clothes on the bed. Then I turned away and gave him some space while I got myself ready to go.

I could see him become more relaxed after that.

Later at the counseling session, we discussed what had happened in the context of understanding how most married couples have different approaches to situations in life, different ways of handling the same events. Dr. Ledford pointed out that our brains are just wired differently. Neither approach is better or worse than the other; they are just different.

He said, "It is like Popeye the Sailor says, 'I yam what I yam.' We all need to accept the differences that we have in these relationships without judging the other person as strange or wrong or less successful in life in some way because they are not like us."

John's LBD intensifies his laidback tendencies. The contrast with my go-getter tendencies increases over time.

Counseling advice like what we received from Dr. Ledford helps me to work with John more on his own terms, which lowers stress for both of us. It makes me a more effective communicator, and John's needs are met more readily. Therefore, my needs get met, too. This is a positive cycle that I hope we can continue with consistency.

28
Handling Urgent Medical Needs

In January 2011, John and I both were sick with a minor virus that drained our energy and attacked our sinuses for a few days. I had asked our local pharmacist if there was anything that might help him with symptoms while we rode it out. The pharmacist said nothing much was effective, but to be careful to watch for secondary infections, especially in the lungs. He said this often happens with patients like John.

I knew he was right, because almost without fail, whenever John would get this kind of thing, he would develop inflammation or infection in his lungs. He has asthma, and it seems to go with that territory. This would happen once or twice a year.

Sure enough, in about four days John was coughing up yellow phlegm. This particular time we ran into two new issues—our two-year-old grandson, Jason, was with us while his family was out of town, and our doctor was not working that day.

Feeling somewhat worried about getting what we needed easily, I called the doctor's office and asked to speak with the nurse. Jackie was sweet, but said the other doctor in the practice required us to come in for a visit before he would prescribe anything. Normally, that would be a reasonable request. The problem was that John was dizzy and very unsteady on his feet. He was also worried about being exposed to any other germs going around during flu/virus season. I said I would try to bring him in.

However, when John tried to get up for a shave and shower, he was not able to stand at the sink and shave. I had to get the shower chair and help him bathe. He was in no shape to move around. And how was I supposed to help him stay balanced and move safely while holding on to little Jason's hand?

I called the doctor's office several times, but got recorded messages. It was frustrating not being able to talk to a person and not being able to get what we needed.

I looked in the medicine cabinet to see if I had any leftover meds that might get John through the day until his regular doctor returned. I found some prednisone. Finally, someone answered at the doctor's office, and I told her I would give John the prednisone, but to please ask Jackie to tell Dr. Dickson about John's condition and request antibiotics for him as usual. She said that it would likely be at least eleven next morning before a prescription would be ready. I asked for an appointment to come in to discuss how to handle it when Dr. Dickson was out of the office in the future, and one was set for a couple of days later.

Next day, no prescription was ready when I called the pharmacy. There were multiple calls again throughout the day culminating in a prescription being picked up around five thirty that afternoon—two days after the first request was made.

The day after that, John and I both went in for the appointment to follow up with Dr. Dickson on how to manage similar situations in the future. She gave us options to deal with these possibilities.

So John and I were both relieved. We felt taken care of again instead of alone and afraid. I hugged her and told her that she was one of the heroes of our story. She told me she admired and respected me for how I take care of John. That meant a lot to me.

I am including this story in my book to encourage caregivers to make that extra appointment with their doctor to discuss options for future stressful event prevention in LBD management.

In my opinion, this is just good medical practice for this disease. The stress causes a lot of physical, mental, and emotional problems for the patient and the caregiver. Some of it is preventable when common sense is applied to the situation.

29
Family Issues and Support

Your world gets smaller when you are caregiving. It feels like the rest of the world is moving on without you. Having friends and family members you can talk to, go places with, vent to, cry with, laugh with, and just be you with is crucial to staying balanced as a caregiver.

During this period of my life, I have come to understand the true value of deep relationships. The folks you thought you wanted as friends sometimes disappear when things get tough, but the ones who are truly there for you stay and dig in with you. You realize what they mean to you and what you mean to them in a whole new way. It is one of the silver linings that comes with a bad diagnosis. Your blessings become very real and deeply wonderful in a strange way.

I think this is why so many people who face tragedy end up saying that it was a blessing. There are insights and understandings that can come in no other way.

To stay connected with others, I have learned to use the phone and the computer for networking when I need emotional support.

Even as she raises two active sons and runs a business, our daughter, Paige, has called us every day. She listens, gives excellent advice, comforts, and encourages me. Paige provides perspective and clarity when I am problem solving and trying to make decisions about the best way to handle a given situation. She knows just what to say and do to calm and love her dad and me and to make us laugh. She comes to visit and invites us to her home often. I cannot say enough about how much she has meant to me throughout this ordeal.

The grandchildren—Michael, Jason, and Nate—are like living Energizer bunnies for me. Their hugs, kisses, and sweet voices recharge my often drained batteries. I just love the way they say my name, "Nana." After a visit with them where I can play with them, read to them, hold them, and just watch them be the sweet little people they are, I feel refreshed. So I drive to see them often and invite them for "one-on-one" visits with Nana and Pop. At the end of their visits with us, I am often physically tired, but my heart and my spirit are full and renewed. With another little grandson on the way, I am looking forward to more love energy in a wonderful new package called grandchild.

My friend, Glenda, has been supportive and loving as well, even though her life is packed with its own responsibilities. My mother has been a sweet daily supporter by phone since she lives five hours away. John's brother, Robert, and his wife, Julie, have invited John to come for visits at their house near Charleston. Those have been especially good times for him, and it has given me a break to have some time when I am not caregiving. Our son, John David, and daughter-in-law, Liz, plan things they know we will like when we visit them. They and my friend, Theresa, are also helping me to edit this book, which is a huge gift of time. Both our children try to be available to go with us to visits with the neurologist, and our son takes notes on his computer while there. All these unselfish acts of kindness have meant so much.

Different friends have provided a variety of help. One takes me out when I am blue or just to do something different, and another brings little goodies by for us. Some make me laugh by sharing funny e-mails. Some provide comic relief just by being who they are. Some share biblical insights that help us or recommend a good book to read, so I can get lost for a while in another world. Some let me help them with their problems, which helps me to feel useful outside my own home and connected with the rest of the world. One gets several of us together every now and then for a girls' trip to the beach. All these things bring me support and loving connections that feed my soul.

There can be a feeling of isolation with any neurological disease and caregiving. People have an initial reaction of concern, and they express how sorry they are that you are dealing with such a bad thing with your loved one. But then there is often a second quiet reaction of retreat emotionally and socially. It is like folks need to have some distance between this monster and themselves. However, when you are the caregiver, you do not have the luxury of this option. You must stay close and remain in the middle of the mix because you are so needed. Fortunately, there are exceptions to this general response. Some people move closer to you to help support you and your loved one, but everyone still has his own life with its own pressures and time constraints.

You may need to be proactive to battle isolation. Sometimes you may need to vent and share your fears and needs. Other times you may need to get away emotionally and just laugh or listen to someone else's problems. Yet again, you may just want to do something for someone who is in a bad situation that will lift his/her burden a little. Reaching out to be involved in all of these activities will help to keep you balanced.

There will likely be some family members and loved ones who do not handle your situation well and whose actions, or lack of action, hurt you. In our family, two of those folks, our son and son-in-law, both of whom initially caused me some pain, have grown as people through their struggle to deal with us in light of the diagnosis, and they are still growing at this point. They have both softened and become more supportive to both John and me as they have dealt with LBD's family impact from their own perspective. Our son has to cope with his own deep grief while helping us cope with ours.

There are two stories that I think need telling because they might help someone else. They both happened in our family. They both are examples of what may happen to you as a caregiver as you and your loved ones struggle to cope with an LBD diagnosis. One is a classic example of when to persevere, and the other is an example of when to let go and let God handle it.

Any time you get a catastrophic diagnosis like LBD in the family, old problems may get exacerbated. You have been traumatized, and you may feel vulnerable and helpless for at least a season of time. You just need more support than usual. As in a construction project, when extra stress is applied, the places most likely to break down are the ones where there are already some problems or where firm connections have yet to be made.

The two stories illustrate how I have coped with the extra stress caused by problems with family members. It is important to say that in both stories, there is love and good intention on the part of everyone. It is also important to say that others in these stories have a different perspective and perhaps even different memories of events.

Learning to communicate effectively and to love unconditionally in a family is difficult to do and maintain over all the changing seasons of life. But we have to still try to do it because the pain from not doing it is not worth it, and the joy from doing it is priceless and irreplaceable.

છ∞ઝ

The first story is about a close family member, whom I will call Joe, and my struggle to deal with the relationship. Joe has unhealed hurts from his childhood when he was molested for years by another family member.

In a family crisis, such as LBD, old hurts in long term relationships can become raw again. I tell this story because there is likely to be someone in your family with whom you have a history that is painful, and the pain drains you when you need every ounce of energy you can get. I suspect this is very common.

My relationship with Joe has been a dramatic roller coaster ride for decades. He would let me come close to him, confide in me, open up, then retreat or lash out in some way. Over the years I always tried to be there for him when he needed anything and even offered to pay for counseling or to go with him. About a year ago he started counseling but did not complete the process to reach a healing of his hurts.

When John was diagnosed with LBD in 2007, at first Joe was supportive in a number of ways, but later he seemed to retreat into the old pattern of disappearing from contact with us for long stretches of time.

Joe's pattern of pulling me in and then pushing me away had always been very painful. I felt rejected and hurt. I told him this, even wrote him letters explaining the pain of his rejections. His responses were unsatisfying, often angry.

When I told Joe that I wanted and needed his support and would appreciate his calls, he said, "Do not expect me to call you. Do not expect it." Those words felt like a punch in the stomach. Much later, when I vented frustration about his long-term pattern of being unavailable even by phone, he blocked me on Facebook. That is sad, and I have had to struggle not to be drained emotionally by his choices.

After weeks of no communication and walking around feeling angry with Joe for his lack of support for me as a caregiver, I decided to discuss the situation with our counselor. Perhaps he could help me cope with the anger and get past it.

I went to see Dr. Ledford alone.

I told him, "I am carrying this person around with me every day in anger and I need to deal with it. My energy is getting drained by this. Can you help me?"

I gave him a synopsis of what had happened on Facebook and reviewed a little of Joe's history and our relationship over the years.

He asked me, "What are the 'shoulds'? What do you think Joe should do?"

I said, "He should answer the phone when I or other family members call him or return that call soon afterward, not ignore it when he is called. He should be a part of helping his mother financially when there is a need and not leave that up to others when it is his responsibility as well. He should give me some emotional support now that I need it, like I have supported him."

Dr. Ledford proceeded to tell me about his little dog that was run over by a car. The dog bit him when he picked it up to take it for medical help. He said, "My dog bit me because it was in pain. I did not get angry with my dog, because I knew his bite was only because he was in pain. Pat, Joe does not bite you because he does not care. Joe bites you because he is in pain."

Tears sprang to my eyes. I knew he was right.

"But I have been bitten over and over again for thirty years. How much more can I take? I have done everything I can think of to help him. What more can I do?"

He said, "There is absolutely nothing you can do. Nothing. You need to get in touch with that. Joe has to want it for himself and do it for himself."

I responded, "I know that in my head, but I have a hard time really living it out. I just want to help him fix it. How can I deal with this?"

He repeated, "Accept that when Joe bites you, it is not because he does not care. It is because he is in pain. Remember that you can do nothing to change him. There is also a block of information you do not have about him at any time. It is like that black box that is sought out after a plane crash with unknown data that can be revealing to what really happened onboard."

Dr. Ledford then explained that people with a history of sexual abuse tend to see themselves as somehow at fault, as "bad."

I said, "Yes, Joe has told me he sees himself as the bad one and me as the good one."

He followed up with, "And Joe resents you for being the good one."

"What in the world do I do with that? Stop doing good things for others?"

"No. Just understand that he does resent you."

I asked him to walk me through what to do again. I needed the repetition. He quietly, patiently did so. I felt my anger draining away somewhat as I walked out of his office. I realized that I needed to just rest in this for a while. It would take time to sink in for good.

At this point in my life I have some big fish to fry. I do not have the energy to fight this fight anymore. I have to give it all to God and to Joe. I cannot fix Joe, probably cannot even help him, but I can love him and pray for him. In a deeper way, I recognize that Joe must do this for himself. It is not up to me. It is up to him.

I may also need to do a version of what I did after Jason was born—let go of the dream I have of the relationship I have always wanted with this person. Perhaps by letting go of that dream, room can be made for new possibilities in both of our lives.

I recently found a beautiful poem written by an unknown author in Jolene Brackey's lovely book, *Creating Moments of Joy.* It describes the healthy choice of letting go for the right reasons.

Let Go

To "let go" does not mean to stop caring;
it means I can't do it for someone else.
To "let go" is not to cut myself off;
it's the realization that I can't control another.
To "let go" is to admit powerlessness,
which means the outcome is not in my hands.
To "let go" is not to try to change or blame another;
it's to make the most of myself.
To "let go" is not to "care for," but to "care about."
To "let go" is not to judge,
but to allow another to be a human being.
To "let go" is not to deny, but to accept.
To "let go" is not to nag, scold, or argue,
but instead to search out my own shortcomings
and correct them.
To "let go" is not to regret the past,
but to grow and live for the future.
To "let go" is to fear less and love more.

Then I must remind myself constantly to focus on those who are there, who have chosen to remain in the orbit of our lives while we move through this journey of darkness.

❧❧❧

The second story is about our son, John David, and me.

John and I made sure when our children, Paige and John David, were small that our first priority would be the family. They grew up in a loving environment, and we were a tight team.

During his last year of high school, John David started to distance himself from us in a number of ways. He rejected our faith as part of his teenage rebellion. Overall, he remained polite and low-key, but he clearly pushed away and wanted distance from us. This stage in his life lasted about ten years.

His early married years were a time of awkward adjustment. It felt like I was held at arm's length when all I wanted to do was hug. There were some uncomfortable exchanges on both sides as we navigated a fitful, frustrating path in trying to communicate better. There was little satisfaction for either of us. It was a strained relationship with sporadic attempts to reconnect that went on for years.

Then came the LBD diagnosis, followed by the meltdown that happened at Paige and Dave's house that I have described earlier. It felt to me like John David supported the notion that we should not move nearby Paige, and that made me feel even more isolated from him as I drove off toward my mother's house on that horrible day. I felt so alone, so helpless, and so vulnerable. That time was the lowest moment of my life. It was black and bleak.

When John David called my mother's house later that night to see if I was there, Mama said, "You are going to have to be the man of the family now. Your mother needs you. She needs your support in this." Her comment was based on watching and listening to my pain about changes in John David over the past ten years as well as the immediate problem.

During their conversation my sister Robin, who was also in the room, hopped up out of her seat, saying, "I can't stand this anymore. I have got to say something."

She did a good job and echoed what Mama had said to him. She also explained what I was feeling and going through, because she had been listening to me as I had laid out all my feelings in Mama's living room, and she knew the history of our relationship.

I vaguely remember getting on the phone with John David. We had a brief conversation.

Then I said, "I'm done."

"What do you mean by that, Mom?"

"I'm just done, John David."

It was a statement of fact. I felt cooked, depleted, hopeless. I could see nothing but my pain.

This statement of mine must have sent some shockwaves through the family. I still have not discussed with John David how that made him feel, but I can imagine that it was not good.

A while after the meltdown, I remember that John David and Liz let me know that they would not be opposed to having John and me live near them as long as there were clear guidelines to protect their privacy, which made perfect sense to me. That was reassuring, and I looked at houses in their area for a few weeks.

But the person I wanted to be closest to was Paige. She was the most supportive and open. She also needed my help with babysitting while she ran their business out of their home. It just made sense to me.

John David has since told me that he and Liz talked over and over about how they could help. I was not aware of his journey at all. He was busy building his IT business in Durham and seemed to have little time to talk to me. He did not share his feelings with me during this time.

He told me that he hated to talk on the phone because he had to talk to people all day in his work. I needed to talk. I needed to talk to my children. But it felt like talking to him violated his space, so I finally stopped trying unless he would call and seemed in the mood to talk. Those times felt few and far between.

When I visited his home, he told me to soften my voice; I was too loud, and I used too many words to say things. Many times he would ask me to stop telling a story because I was taking too long and giving too many details. So I stopped going much at all, and when I did go, I stayed briefly. When I was there, I was always afraid of being criticized again. It felt like I was out of place and intruding on their peace and quiet—someone who was endured rather than enjoyed.

The contrast with going to Paige's house was huge. There I was literally greeted with big smiles and warm hugs and even cheers from little Michael, who was not quite two years old. There I was Nana—wanted, needed, even adored. My name was spoken with soft, loving tones, and my singing, dancing, and laughter were applauded and enjoyed. Dave had apologized for the tone of his reaction on the day of my meltdown, and we were working on our relationship.

When Jason, Paige's second son, was born in 2008, the lovefest continued at her house. Nana was needed, appreciated, loved, and totally in love with those grandsons. I had a purpose there and visited often to help Paige as she juggled working and keeping up with two little ones.

Even after John David's son, Nate, was born in January 2009, things did not improve that much. None of us knew Nate's name until he was born. Liz and John David decided to keep that to themselves. I still felt held at arm's length. My visits were short at their house, and their visits to our house were twice a year and seemed to always get abbreviated from the original plan. I had trouble feeling like I could just relax and be myself with them. I think I felt unliked.

All throughout these years, I was trying to reach out and make the communication better and deeper. I wanted an adult friendship with John David and to feel comfortable in his presence again. We would have some meaningful sharing, and then something would distance us again. He always seemed too busy or too tired to take the time to invest in the relationship. I heard those two excuses over and over again.

"I'm just exhausted, Mom. It has been a tough week." Or "I cannot listen to any more words. I have to listen to people all day, and I am just burned out." These words were said in many phone calls when I wanted to catch him up on what was happening to his dad or to problem solve some issue. He simply was not available much of the time.

One way I tried to create a time for us to just sit and talk was on my birthday each year. When he would ask me what I wanted for my birthday, I would say, "I want you to take me out for a wonderful dinner for the evening—just you and me."

At first he did not understand, but then he agreed, and we continue to do that every year.

On my birthday in 2009, he took me to an Italian restaurant. As we ate, he began to talk about improving our relationship. He shared that he felt trapped between Liz and me and wanted us to learn how to relate better to one another. He also was clear that he knew it was going to happen eventually, but he wanted it sooner rather than later. He asked me what Liz could do to make me feel more welcome in their home.

I said, "She could smile at me when she sees me at the door. She could hug me."

I did not enjoy that birthday dinner much. The conversation was heavy, and I felt somewhat corrected again. At the end of the evening, I was down, but I later realized that it was a breakthrough event. John David had opened up and admitted that he wanted things to be much better just like I did.

From that point on, Liz and I both worked hard to sense what we could do to make each other feel comfortable. She smiled and gave me a warm hug the next time I visited their house. That felt wonderful. I brought some of my own food with me for my visits, because their taste in food was different from mine. Liz would have those foods in her refrigerator the next time I would visit, letting me know she was trying to meet my needs. I could tell she was trying, and it made me love her more.

After Nate was a few months old, John David began to ask me to stay overnight at his house. He even gave me a gift of coupons for multiple night stays with them to encourage me to spend more time with them. He was clearly reaching out to me, but I was so easily hurt by his "corrections" of the way I talked and acted at his house that it was painful for me to be there for any length of time. I explained all this to him several times.

I finally said, "Stop correcting me. I am your mother."

But over time I tried to enter their house quietly, even whispering, and to give them condensed versions of any stories I told. It was hard for me to do that every time, though. I wanted them to know what I was experiencing and feeling or to give them background information so they would understand why I had made a certain choice about John's care, but they seemed not so interested in the details. They made it clear they wanted the short version.

John David tried to call more often, but he still struggles with doing that. I tried to use Facebook and e-mail to communicate more since they both seem to prefer that to the phone.

Another breakthrough was the first time Nate was left overnight alone with us at our house. He did very well, and we all had a good time. Nate was a happy camper when they returned. That seemed to make them feel more at ease.

John David now takes Friday off from work to allow for a longer weekend visit at our house. It gives him more time to decompress from a hectic workweek, and he is more present with us when he is rested.

Over time we have all worked to find out what each of us needs from the other and to accommodate those needs as quickly as possible. We still often do not agree on religion or politics, but we do agree on our love and support for each other. The result is that we are closer and much more at peace with one another.

જી૦ડ

Both these stories are still ongoing. Hopefully, both will ultimately have a happy ending. They are examples of how life goes on as caregiving happens. Opportunities to grow as people within the context of difficult circumstances present themselves, perhaps with greater boldness, in the midst of our darker journeys in life.

30
Bobcats and Turtles

During a session with our counselor, Dr. Terry Ledford, we were talking about the differences in the way people approach emotional issues in their lives.

Dr. Ledford said at one point in the discussion, "Think about the bobcat. When it is confronted with some perceived threat or challenge, what is its response? It shows its teeth and claws and moves forward. It asserts its strength to fight the threat.

"The response of the turtle to the same thing makes absolutely no sense to the bobcat. The turtle withdraws inside of its shell. It retreats from the perceived challenge or threat. Turtles want distance from the perceived threat."

I am including these comments from our counselor because I suspect that in any family dealing with a diagnosis of LBD, there are going to be family members who respond differently to the threat and challenge that comes with the diagnosis. The primary caregiver is going to have to deal with all of these responses in a way that allows you to keep your own balance. If you lose your balance, things can get bad very quickly.

Some of us are bobcats, and some of us are turtles. All of us care when a loved one is in crisis. Just knowing that has helped me keep my balance.

Learning the art of dealing with both types of people is not easy. It is ongoing. I am getting better at it over time. Here is what I understand so far.

Bobcats are more assertive, even aggressive at times. They use more words and tend to be verbally expressive. They are more direct and confrontational in their thinking and speech, and their default response to hurt, fear, or frustration is anger. They have problems with feelings of rejection.

Turtles are somewhat more passive with their emotions. They use fewer words in general and struggle with expression of their feelings. They like to "go in a cave," so to speak and avoid or escape confrontation. They like some distance in their relationships. They have a "live and let live" mindset and assume things will often work out on their own. Their default response to hurt, fear, or frustration is silence or retreat. They have problems with criticism.

Married couples are often one of each. To improve communication and satisfaction in the relationship, each person must do some work to change his normal pattern.

Bobcats have to learn to approach situations more softly, less confrontationally. The number of words needs to be reduced with simultaneous reduction of volume and intensity. They also need to be careful of sounding critical and figure out how to say what is needed softly. If bobcats feel anger, they should seek out within themselves the hurt, fear, or frustration underneath that anger and give the hurt, fear, or frustration a soft voice. When these feelings are addressed appropriately, the anger will dissipate. Their anger response is viewed by the turtle as criticism.

Turtles have to learn to use more words in general and especially in the expression of emotions. They need to put their hurts, fears, or frustrations into words. They have to fight the urge to retreat into their shell and stay in the conversation or situation until it is resolved. Their retreat is viewed by the bobcat as rejection.

Learning to break the patterns of the bobcat and the turtle is not easy, and it takes time. It does yield good fruit though, and it is worth the effort.

The good news is that when one person in the relationship chooses to change his own pattern, there can be improvement overall. That is because the communication pattern for bobcats and turtles is circular.

For example, if the bobcat gets better at softening speech, the turtle is less likely to go into his shell. The less the turtle goes into his shell, the less rejection is felt by the bobcat, who then is less critical of the turtle. A positive spiral can replace the former negative one.

John and I have worked on improving our pattern of communication, and the difference is huge in our relationship. The stress of caregiving is greatly reduced for me. But I have also learned to apply some of this to other relationships and seen the benefits there as well.

31
Where We Are Now

We have been blessed to get an early diagnosis for John, but it does not feel early at all to me. It has been going on for years for us.

Five years after diagnosis, John has a much smaller stride. His arms no longer swing at all when he walks. He leans when he stands and is developing a slumped posture. Visual-spatial issues are a problem. He no longer drives.

His memory is often excellent for many things most days, but he can forget what was said 10–30 minutes ago on a bad day. His initiative and stamina are poor. He has trouble with multiple directions for things and likes to be told one thing at a time.

He has some trouble getting dressed. He gets dizzy sometimes and falls on occasion, and he does not handle loud places or lots of people well. On a bad day, he can be irritable, difficult, and argumentative, maybe even a little paranoid. John can say things that make no sense until I dig a little and "connect the dots." It is like he is speaking out in the middle of a story going on in his head.

But he remains alert and able to engage with family and friends as he enjoys his daily life.

We are very thankful for the loved ones who have given such close and vital support to us. Some call every day to check on us.

We appreciate the medical team who are helping us through the maze of LBD. It was worth the time and effort to find medical professionals who are good listeners, good practitioners, and just good people. Compassionate care that includes the caregiver is a huge help in dealing with this disease.

Somehow in the process of walking in this painful place, we have grown. We have indeed found treasures in the darkness. We have worked hard, knowing our time is not endless together. We love each other more and our whole family communicates much better now—more honestly, more freely, and more deeply. We are kinder and gentler than we were before, and we are stronger in a quiet way. We appreciate the sweetness of days together. We are learning to let go of things we cannot change and things that do not matter. We are learning to live in the moment.

These are no small things.

A diagnosis such as LBD feels like the end of everything at first. But it is really the beginning of a new journey—not one we want to make, but the journey has a purpose. And there are still good days and times ahead.

There are actually treasures in the darkness that you may find along the way. I know. I have found some of them. I plan to keep looking.

Early Stage LBD Caregiving Tips

Controlling Stressors
Managing Medicine and Supplements
Working with Medical Professionals
Making the House Work for You
Taking Care of Yourself
Getting Enough Sleep
Social support
Counseling
Love
Faith
Travel
Eating
Exercise
Massage Therapy
Preserving Personhood
Brain-Building Activities
Dealing with the Unexpected
Putting Your Legal Ducks in a Row

∞⁂∞

Notice the shape of the tips list. It is an hourglass to remind me of the importance of time.

Every day is precious; every moment to be cherished. Living in the moment that is now, and making it count, is a secret to happiness in this walk.

Do not dwell in the past—you cannot change it. Do not dwell in the future—it may never come or may be different from your predictions. Dwell and focus on now.

The frustration of LBD is that what works for one may not work for another. The beauty of LBD is what may not work for one may work for your loved one. The challenge of LBD is finding what works for your loved one and continuing to tweak it.

Hopefully, some of these tips will make it easier for you and your loved one to navigate through early stage LBD, maybe even finding some treasures of your own along the way.

Controlling Stressors

I have become convinced over time that controlling stress is a key to managing the early stage of this disease. When things are calm or my response to a fear, hurt, worry, or frustration is soft toward John, everything works better. The day is sweeter, and John's physical symptoms seem to be better.

My first tip is one that has worked for me over and over again.

- **Choose the lesser stressor** when there is an option for how to do something.
- Eliminate people from your daily routine who will drag you down emotionally, and add people who "get it."
- Learn to say no. You already have a huge job and ministry to do.
- Prioritize what you need to do in your day and try to work that plan.
- Choose the important over the urgent.
- Ignore negative people and comments. They will drain you of energy you need.
- Laugh every chance you get. Be with those who bring you laughter.
- Make time for yourself to recharge your batteries. Do some things you really like to do.

- Exercise.
- Organize your financial matters to simplify when and where you pay your bills and handle your investments.
- Simplify everything you can.
- Pay for what you cannot or should not do.
- Leave guilt behind.
- Pray.

Managing Medicine and Supplements

Management of medicines is a huge part of good caregiving. The right medicine taken at the right time can make a big difference in the quality of the day, but the wrong medicine or medicine taken at the wrong time can create a disaster with LBD. Patients with this disease can be very sensitive to the wrong medication or even to a moderate dose of the right medication.

My understanding from John's neurologist is that almost any new medicine should be started at a low dosage and slowly increased until it is effective for that particular patient. He says to start one new medicine at a time, so there is only that one pharmacological variable to consider if a change occurs in the patient.

I am not a medical person, but as John's caregiver, I feel an obligation to find out how to protect him from unnecessary harm. From my research of various sources, I have collected some names of medicines that may cause problems if your loved one has LBD. Some of them have the potential to cause irreversible and significant damage to an LBD patient. If you have not already done so, read the foreword in this book by Dr. Daniel Kaufer. In it he discusses the heightened sensitivity to various drugs that occurs with LBD.

A *Beware of Possible Adverse Effects List* may act as an informal alert system to use with medical professionals to get them to stop and do their own appropriate research before taking action that could cause harm. None of the lists included here should be considered as definitive or complete. There will always be variations among patients due to the complexity of this disease. Sometimes with some patients, a medicine listed here may help and not cause harm. I doubt that any such list would ever be complete for every LBD patient. **It is merely a guide to assist you as a caregiver and hopefully help avoid some bad outcomes by allowing a wise question to be asked at the right time.**

The first group of drugs to add to your *Beware List* is more of a category of drugs and is included on the Medical Alert Wallet Card created by the LBDA. For emergency treatment of psychosis, it advises avoidance of traditional or typical antipsychotic agents, such as Haldol (haloperidol). It states that newer atypical antipsychotic agents, such as quetiapine (Seroquel) and clozapine (Clozaril), should be used at the lowest possible dose and with caution. It warns that some of the traditional antipsychotics can cause permanent, irreversible, or even fatal reactions. The card contains some guidance for ER personnel as they treat the LBD patient. Copies of this wallet card may be found on the LBDA Web site. On the home page, search for "wallet card." Also on the LBDA Web site is a more comprehensive physician's guide to treating LBD patients with behavioral disturbances. It can be found at the following web address, www.lbda.org/go/ER, which is also given on the wallet card.

The second group of drugs to add to the *Beware List* is from John's neurologist, Dr. Daniel Kaufer, who has served on the LBDA Scientific Advisory Council. Drugs that block the action of acetylcholine, a brain chemical involved in attention and memory processes, may cause confusion and hallucinations in LBD patients. However, there may be circumstances where drugs in this class may be more beneficial, as for example, in maintaining urinary bladder control. But as I understand it, a good rule of thumb is to be wary of these anticholinergic medications. Remember, you should always consult the doctor who is most familiar with a particular patient's situation for advice on what medicines will work for your loved one. None of the information in this book is intended to replace your doctor's medical advice.

Medicines with anticholinergic effects (most anticholinergic first)

- Atropine (100 percent of maximal anticholinergic effect)
- Scopolamine
- Tolterodine
- Hyoscyamine
- Cholinergic Parkinsonism agents
- Trihexyphenidyl
- Benztropine
- Diphenhydramine (Benadryl)
- Amitriptyline (Elavil)
- Digoxin
- Nifedipine
- Phenobarbital
- Oxybutynin (20 percent)
- Isosorbide dinitrate
- Hydroxyzine
- Warfarin
- Dipyridamole
- Codeine
- Ranitidine (10 percent)

- Dyazide
- Furosemide (Lasix)
- Nortriptyline

Other medicines to add to the *Beware List* might include Phenergan (promethazine), Reglan (metoclopramide), and Compazine (prochlorperazine), all of which are used for treating nausea. Reglan is also used for heartburn caused by acid reflux. Phenergan is also used before and after surgery to help relax patients and to treat allergies. Compazine is also used to treat vertigo and migraines.

For anesthesia, one research study in 2007 at the University of Pittsburg School of Medicine suggested that certain types of anesthesia may be more or less risky. You may want to research that information for yourself on the Internet before any surgery.

Other good resources for information about medicines to avoid are found in *A Caregiver's Guide to Lewy Body Dementia* by Helen Buell Whitworth and James A. Whitworth and *Living With Lewy's* by Amy and Gerald Throop. Both of these books provide a comprehensive look at LBD caregiving through all the stages of the disease and should be part of your library as an LBD caregiver.

As always, your own research and your own physician, especially a good LBD specialist, is your best resource. None of my recommendations qualify as medical advice. I am simply a caregiver, like you, who has tried to find information to trigger intelligent discussions with medical professionals who might come in contact with my husband. My goal has been to get them to research and think carefully before giving John any medicine that might cause him harm.

The following tips involve general management of medicines with the LBD patient.

- Be in charge of dispensing medicine at home. This is not negotiable.
- Keep the LBDA Medical Alert Card with you.
- Keep a list in your wallet of possible medicines to avoid, and use it to prompt discussion and research.
- Avoid the emergency room if you can.
- Make a chart of medicines and supplements. Make separate columns for each time of day they are taken. Include strengths of each one.
- Use the chart when you sort pills each week into a pill box.
- Keep the chart with prescription bottles in a container so everything is in one place.
- Bring the medicines chart to all medical appointments.
- Make a list of prescriptions that need refilling before your next appointment.
- Use the Internet to find possible conflicts for medicines and supplements. Make adjustments with help of pharmacist and doctor.
- Familiarize yourself with trade and generic names of medicines.
- Be alert to new studies that address LBD, and discuss these with your doctors.
- Request a new prescription if the doctor increases the number of pills to be taken in a day.
- Keep a history of medicines that did not work well for your loved one.
- Ask for timed release versions of medicines to simplify your schedule and to provide more consistent effects.
- Ask the pharmacist if any medicines are available in a ninety-day supply and get prescriptions for those.
- Use one pharmacy if you can.
- Consult a geriatric pharmacist for guidance.

- Coordinate all prescriptions to be filled on the same day of the month with help from your pharmacist.
- Do only one thing at a time in terms of addressing symptoms or treatment.
- Start new medicines slowly and watch for negative side effects.

Working with Medical Professionals

- If you have any reservations about diagnosis, treatment philosophy, or communication with any doctor, always seek a second opinion.
- Do not stop looking for the right doctor until you find a match for you as well as your loved one. You need care, too.
- Make sure it is easy to contact and get a response from doctors in a timely manner. I use e-mail with one and phone with the other.
- Choose your battles. Contact the doctor for important issues only, and try to solve the lesser issues yourself until your next appointment.
- On the other hand, call before a problem becomes a crisis.
- Make a written list of questions or issues you need to discuss for your appointment times.
- Make a copy of your question list for you and for the doctor.
- Use your copy to take notes as the doctor responds to your questions so you will remember it all later.
- Date your notes and file them in a folder that you can easily find later.

- Take someone with you to doctor appointments to help you remember what to ask and what is said and to take notes.
- Always have the LBDA.org card with you to alert ER folks of the LBD diagnosis and medicines that can do great harm.
- Take a copy of the *Beware List* with you to medical appointments as you and the doctor weigh benefits versus side effects.
- Contact your local palliative care providers, who have the goal of improving quality of life by relieving symptoms of disease. They may help you coordinate your medical team approach to LBD and give you emotional support and guidance.
- Give a list to each health care provider of all the other providers caring for your loved one.
- Take a copy of the "What is LBD?" page from the LBDA Web site (www.lbda.org) to any new doctor.
- Prepare a bag for medical emergencies. Include medicine chart, change of clothes, wipes, Depends, something to read, and snacks.
- Once again, avoid the emergency room if you can.

Making the House Work for You

- Think of home improvements as good investments to delay nursing home entry and improve quality of life.
- Invest in making external and internal doorways senior friendly.
- Have ramps or cement inclines built where needed. Be creative and make them pretty as well as functional to add value to your home.
- Make sure lighting is good all over the house.
- Get motion sensitive LED lights to light the way to the bathroom after dark.
- Eliminate clutter and create visual order. Put things in their place and return them there when you finish with them.
- Move furniture that blocks traffic areas.
- Remove area rugs that could slip and cause falls.
- Get in a borrowed wheelchair yourself and maneuver around your house to see where potential problem areas exist. Modify those areas.
- Have someone come every other week to clean your home if you can afford it.

• If you live in a split-level or split-foyer house or if all bedrooms are on the second floor, move if you can to a one-level house.

For the Bathroom:
• Remodel the bathroom early to create a wet zone and drain for the tiled bathroom floor.
• If complete bathroom remodeling is not an option, then modify the bath area by installing a step-in shower.
• Modify the toilet area with a wall hung or handicapped height toilet.
• Invest in a toilet bidet seat.
• Install handgrips everywhere you need them.
• Use a handheld showerhead with a push button option for water flow reduction.
• Tile any area that may be impacted by water.
• Use small floor tiles for a better gripping surface.
• Buy a comfortable, sturdy shower chair.
• Make your remodel project as attractive as possible.
• Install a motion sensitive overhead light.

Taking Care of Yourself

It is essential that you take care of yourself in the process of caregiving. If you collapse, your loved one will collapse as well. So it is not selfish to sometimes put yourself first in your choices as a caregiver.

Here are some strategies that can make you a better caregiver:

- Have some physical activity each day.
- Stay in the moment as much as possible.
- Take a couple of long, slow, deep breaths when you feel stressed.
- Keep up to date on your medical and dental appointments.
- Take your own medicines on time each day.
- Eat well.
- Stay hydrated.
- Ask your doctor for a prescription for anxiety to be taken only when you need it.
- Treat yourself with something you like to eat, drink, or do.
- Stay connected with friends and family and be open about what you are going through.
- Take breaks.
- Be aware of your limits when lifting or moving your loved one.

- Reduce and manage clutter.
- Accept help when it is offered. Prepare a list of what you need ahead of time.
- Keep your appearance neat.
- Decorate for holidays.
- Refuse to feel guilty.
- Keep a journal or diary. Writing can be cathartic.
- Keep some creative project nearby for stimulation and escape from routine.
- Do something intellectually stimulating like reading or puzzles each day, even if it is brief.
- Buy a yoga video and try it.
- Close your eyes and visualize yourself in a peaceful spot.
- Find someone or something to make you laugh. Laughter is wonderful medicine for the soul.

Getting Enough Sleep

- As soon as possible after LBD diagnosis, ask the doctor to address sleep issues as part of the treatment plan if sleep disorders are present in the patient.
- Do only one thing at a time in terms of addressing sleep symptoms or treatment.
- Find a doctor who will allow you as caregiver to communicate as needed with him/her to fine-tune all treatments for maximum results.
- Be sure to get enough sleep yourself.
- Try melatonin first.

Social Support

- Let people know how you feel and what you need. Be open and honest.
- Use the telephone for brief conversations with friends and relatives in town and out of town.
- Use e-mail and social network sites on the Internet.
- Write notes and send cards to others who are in need or who have a special event to celebrate.
- Visit your local senior center to see what kinds of activities you and your loved one can enjoy with others.
- Go to church if you are not already doing so. Join a Sunday school class or Bible study there.
- Attend a meeting of any support group that fits your situation.
- Invite friends out to lunch or have them over to your house. Keep the menu simple and easy to do.
- Invite friends for coffee.
- If you have friends over, buy a small bouquet of flowers at your grocery store. When you walk past it later, you will be reminded of the sweet sharing time you just had with them.
- Seek out people who need something you can provide. Give them that gift of your time and self.
- Stay connected to others.

- Welcome new friends into your life.
- Find people who are wrestling with similar problems who will understand.
- Find people who are not wrestling with similar problems to help you get your mind off your issues.
- Try to keep your focus on those who care about you.

Counseling

- Find a good counselor that both of you trust.
- If the first counselor is not a match for you, keep looking.
- Ask the counselor to keep in mind that controlling your loved one's stress level is paramount in the process of counseling.
- Be open and honest about all issues.
- Be humble enough to admit when you are the one who needs to change. Without this, no counseling will ever help you.
- Bring whatever is bothering you at the time to the attention of the counselor.
- Do what the counselor recommends.

Love

One of the strange gifts that can come with LBD and other degenerative neurological diseases is the keen awareness of the preciousness of each day. Our time together is not taken for granted. It is cherished. John and I are both conscious at this stage of the disease of how important it is to build strong, loving memories.

- Figure out how to express love to each other in the way the other person can understand and receive it. Do this early and often.
- Get counseling to help you learn to better communicate, express love, and find peace.
- Consciously make good memories together.
- Use words.
- Use touch.
- Practice kindness in all things.
- Be quick to ask forgiveness when you are wrong and to give it when you are right.

Faith

- Do not ask God, "Why?"
- Ask God, "How do I grow in this?"
- Ask God, "What are you teaching me in this? What are the lessons?"
- Ask others to pray for you and your loved one.
- Pray for others and seek ways to help them.
- Keep praying for joy, insight, wisdom, and strength.
- Read your Bible expectantly every day for guidance and strength.
- Stay connected to fellow believers.
- Seek God's best in each day, and dwell on the positives.
- Admit your weaknesses and give them to God.
- Give God those things you cannot control anyway.
- Praise God by singing out loud to Him.

Travel

A good rule of thumb in deciding whether to make a big trip is to trust your own instincts about it. Will it help and enrich you and your loved one, or will it likely hurt?

- Plan ahead, making choices based on current physical needs.
- If flying, choose a location that offers a nonstop flight if possible.
- When making reservations indicate the need for handicapped services.
- Use a wheelchair if there is any fatigue or stress. It will put you in front of every line.
- If this is your last big vacation, tell key people and ask for upgrades.
- Select low-stress activities for both of you.
- Do something for yourself on this trip that is a special treat to energize or pamper you.
- Rent that convertible. It will be worth every extra penny to have the experience and the memory!

Eating

- Eat a Mediterranean diet with fresh veggies, fish, olive oil, and red wine if there is no conflict with medicines.
- Set up your plate so it is half green or bright veggies, one-fourth lean protein, one-fourth starch.
- Add organic, extra virgin coconut oil to your diet every day. It may provide an alternate source of energy for brain cells.
- Shop the perimeter of the store avoiding processed foods.
- Splurge occasionally to add some fun to life.

Exercise

Generally speaking, the earlier you address issues, the longer you may retain normal or close to normal function. Studies show exercise can increase new brain connections by a factor of four.

- Buy some exercise equipment that you can have at home for ease and frequency of use.
- If you cannot purchase equipment, join a local gym and go regularly.
- Use yoga DVDs for beginners or seniors to learn basic stretches.
- Use a tool like the Dyna-Disc to improve balance.
- Ask your doctor to give you a prescription for physical therapy as soon as any movement symptoms appear after diagnosis.
- Use two-pound weights in/on each hand/wrist to walk around the house. For some reason, this sometimes restores stride to normal levels.
- Seek out DVDs that can help with specific exercises at home.
- Consider hiring a personal trainer to go with your loved one to physical therapy and help follow up at home with appropriate exercises.

Massage Therapy

John fell while visiting his brother Robert. He injured his right shoulder so that the use of his arm diminished significantly. Over time I noticed that he had practically stopped using the right arm for simple tasks, such as picking up a glass.

Chiropractic adjustments seemed to help a little, and then I added visits with a massage therapist. Vicki Bates, a sensitive, caring woman and excellent massage therapist, worked on John using deep therapeutic massage to help restore his ability to lift his arm and to get him to use the arm again in a more normal way. He can now lift his right arm without any pain, which he could not do for months before seeing her. Unfortunately, he had gotten out of the habit of using this arm. He has learned to use it again for the most part, but still not like before.

Vicky also works on his feet and legs to stretch and relax muscles and restore some more fluidity in his stride.

- Find a massage therapist to work on keeping muscles stretched and more relaxed.
- Go yourself as well.

Preserving Personhood

John's neurologist, Dr. Kaufer, has told us that his goal is "preserving personhood" for his LBD patients. Those words are golden for me. They speak volumes about who Dr. Kaufer is as a physician and a man. He understands the power of hope and feeling some level of control when faced with a challenge like LBD. He is always available to us via e-mail.

John's primary care physician, Dr. Lori Dickson, meets us at every appointment with alert, gentle ears and eyes. She laughs with us and makes us feel that we are important to her as she evaluates what is needed at every juncture of John's care. She uses common sense as she manages his condition and is one of the best listeners I have encountered in the medical profession.

John's psychologist, Dr. Terry Ledford, is an artful and sensitive practitioner. He has kept faithfully my request that John's stress level be kept low as he has navigated us both through channels of deeper communication. His skills have not only preserved personhood for John, but have taught John how to express that personhood more freely and openly. I believe that he has actually created more space and time for John to enjoy life by giving us both tools to know and understand each other better.

Finding doctors such as these, who understand not only the science of a disease, but the treatment that will preserve and protect the humanity and social well-being of the patient, is hard to do. But it is worth the time and effort it takes to build the medical support team that will manage our lives during this journey.

Preserving personhood means getting the right medical care, but also addressing issues that might steal independence or take away from simple pleasures. Sometimes it means pushing John a little beyond where he wants to go to keep him more active.

LBD attacks your clarity of thought, your memory, your ability to take care of your basic physical needs, your social interactions with others, your balance, and your ability to move normally. How you see others and how you appear to them change over time, but also in a fluctuating way within a day or from day to day. Maintaining your own personhood for as long as possible is such an important part of treating the symptoms of this disease.

- Find doctors who believe in the concept of preserving personhood.
- Be an active team coordinator of these medical professionals.
- Protect your loved one from too much stress.
- Encourage your loved one to stay as involved and active for as long as possible in things that he loves.
- Be willing and humble enough to do what you have to do to grow as a caregiver and person.

Brain Building Activities

- Use any game that includes recall, sorting, organizing, computing, or other brain workouts.
- Play card games with friends to combine social stimulation with brain exercise.
- Dance to combine socializing, balance, and movement.
- Invest in a tool such as the iPad for brain exercise apps that are portable and easy to use.
- Take advantage of free services such as Talking Books to continue the stimulation of reading. Phone the National Library Service for the Blind and Physically Handicapped for their talking book digital machine at 1-888-NLS-READ or use their Web site at www.gov/nls.
- Exercise to enhance brain building.
- Use the AARP Web site for free games.
- Find other Internet options by searching for "brain games for seniors" or "brain fitness."
- Play Password. You can buy used games on Ebay and Amazon.
- Modify and simplify game rules as needed.

Dealing with the Unexpected

Some days John will just be difficult. Or we may be having a perfectly normal day, I enter the room, and he is seething and lashes out at me unexpectedly. This is part of LBD for John. It fluctuates without warning.

Learning to deal effectively with this is an ongoing process for me. It will likely be different for each caregiver and patient. Sometimes I react with resentment and anger and have to come back and apologize later. Sometimes I react calmly and gently. With John, the calmer, quieter approach seems to work better. Occasionally, I have to firmly react to him to get him to stop and break the cycle. Mostly, I play it by ear and ask God to guide me in the right approach for that particular time.

It is important to share information with the neurologist if aggressiveness or moodiness is becoming more frequent. These symptoms may need to be addressed with medication if they become frequent or too intense.

If you are not in counseling, this is an avenue you might pursue with your loved one. If he refuses to go with you or is too sick to respond well, you go and get some help with coping skills for yourself. Sometimes for us, just learning to express what we are really feeling out loud to each other has diffused a lot of emotion and calmed the waters at home. It sounds simple, but it has worked for us many times.

- Try the calm, gentle, quiet approach if your loved one gets feisty.
- Leave the room and return later for a fresh start.
- To diffuse irrational anger agree with him that he is right and you are wrong.
- Check with the neurologist if mood variance symptoms get worse.
- Get into counseling to add some more coping skills to your set of tools.

Putting Your Legal Ducks in a Row

If you have not already done so, basic legal documents should be created for both you and your loved one during the early stage of LBD. Be sure that anyone designated to make decisions for you or for your loved one is aware of this designation, is in agreement with it, has good communication with you, and is fully aware of your wishes.

- Get a will as soon as possible.
- Get a Durable Power of Attorney as soon as possible.
- Get a Health Care Power of Attorney as soon as possible to avoid expensive and draining guardianship proceedings.
- Research what other legal documents may be required in your area and get the appropriate signatures for those. Have them in place in advance of when they may be needed.
- Contact all insurance companies early and find out how you can become the contact person in case your loved one is not able to speak for himself.

*Seek first the kingdom of God and His righteousness, and all
these things shall be added unto you. Therefore do not worry
about tomorrow, for tomorrow will worry about itself.*
Matthew 6:33–34

Resources That Have Helped Me

www.lbda.org

This Web site focuses on LBD, giving background information, current research, and opportunities to connect with other LBD caregivers. It was the first place recommended to me by John's neurologist.

www.caring.com

This Web site addresses the needs of caregivers for all types of diseases. I have found it to be very practical, interesting, and helpful.

www.caregiver.org

This Web site is the Family Caregiver Alliance, which has excellent information about LBD. Type "LBD" into their search box to find it.

www.eldercare.gov

This is the government Web site sponsored by the Administration on Aging. You will find much information on how to access local support. There is also a good caregiver tips section.

A Caregiver's Guide to Lewy Body Dementia by Helen Buell Whitworth, MS, BSN, and James A. Whitworth, 2010

This is a comprehensive and instructive guide for the LBD caregiver written by one of the founders of the LBDA. It is well written and very informative.

Living With Lewy's; Empowering Today's Dementia Caregiver by Amy and Gerald Throop, 2010
This is another comprehensive and instructive guide that is chocked full of detailed and practical helps and tips for any dementia caregiver.

Creating Moments of Joy by Jolene Brackey, 2007
Jolene Brackey works with Alzheimer's and dementia patients and teaches others how to do this more positively in her educational seminars. Her "can do" approach of enriching life for patients is infectious and powerful. The book is full of simple and practical ways to create moments of joy for others with short term memory loss and has journal spaces for the reader to add what works specifically with your own loved one.

Precious Lord, Take My Hand by Shelly Beach, 2007
This is a Christian devotional book designed for caregivers. The author has been a caregiver for multiple family members and shares meaningful, pertinent lessons she has learned along with biblical insights that offer encouragement.

Life in the Balance: A Physician's Memoir of Life, Love, and Loss with Parkinson's Disease and Dementia by Thomas Graboys, MD and Peter Zheutlin, 2008
This memoir gives insight into what it is like to be a patient with LBD and Parkinson's disease.

Acknowledgements

Many people have helped to make this book possible.

Dr. Daniel Kaufer, MD, is Director of UNC Memory Disorders Clinic and Division Chief of Cognitive Neurology and Memory Disorders at UNC. He suggested that I write the book and graciously offered to write the foreword for it. This encouraged me to persevere and complete the task. His caring practice of medicine has offered hope in our journey.

Dr. Terry Ledford, PhD, is a practicing psychologist in Rutherfordton, NC. He gave us tools to uncover treasures we may never have found without his help.

Dr. Lori Dickson, MD, her compassionate staff, and the wonderful people at Smith's Drug Store have made life calm and gentle enough for me to get this book written and edited over the past two years. Our medical team has made a huge difference for us.

John David Snyder and Liz Snyder spent hours editing and going over the content of our story, the tips section, and selection of the cover photo, which he photographed. As they read and we all discussed the story, our love deepened for each other.

My lifelong friend, Theresa Dice, did intensive editing. My mother, Marjorie Overman, and friends, Glenda Jowers and Jane

McCall, edited for appropriate content and presentation. How can you thank friends who give of themselves so freely?

No one person has given like our daughter, Paige Telep, through every step of our journey. There are not enough hugs or thank yous to cover her generosity of spirit.

Last, but not least, my beloved John encouraged me as I wrote it, listened as I read the book to him, and then gave his nod of approval.

May God bless you all for your kindness.

This Irish Blessing
has been a part of every big moment in our lives.

May the road rise to meet you.
May the wind be always at your back.
May the sun shine warm upon your face,
The rains fall softly on your fields.
And until we meet again,
May God hold you in the palm of His hand.

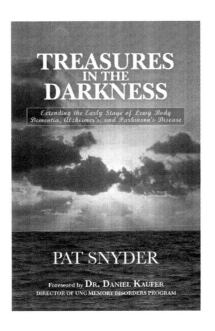

If you would like to share your comments with the author of *Treasures in the Darkness,* you can do so at her email address, patsnyder137@gmail.com, facebook.com/Treasuresinthedarkness, or her blog, http://lbd-caregiver.blogspot.com.

Made in the USA
Lexington, KY
25 May 2012